About the Fraser Institute

The Fraser Institute is an independent Canadian economic and social research and educational organization. It has as its objective the redirection of public attention to the role of competitive markets in providing for the well-being of Canadians. Where markets work, the Institute's interest lies in trying to discover prospects for improvement. Where markets do not work, its interest lies in finding the reasons. Where competitive markets have been replaced by government control, the interest of the Institute lies in documenting objectively the nature of the improvement or deterioration resulting from government intervention.

The Fraser Institute is a national, federally-chartered, non-profit organization financed by the sale of its publications and the tax-deductible contributions of its members, foundations, and other supporters; it receives no government funding.

Editorial Advisory Board

Prof. Armen Alchian
Prof. Jean-Pierre Centi
Prof. Michael Parkin
Prof. L.B. Smith

Prof. J.M. Buchanan
Prof. Herbert G. Grubel
Prof. Friedrich Schneider
Sir Alan Walters

Senior Fellows

Murray Allen, MD
Dr. Paul Brantingham
Prof. Barry Cooper
Prof. Herb Emery
Gordon Gibson
Prof. Ron Kneebone
Dr. Owen Lippert
Prof. Jean-Luc Migue
Dr. Filip Palda

Prof. Eugene Beaulieu
Martin Collacott
Prof. Steve Easton
Prof. Tom Flanagan
Dr. Herbert Grubel
Prof. Rainer Knopff
Prof. Ken McKenzie
Prof. Lydia Miljan
Prof. Chris Sarlo

Adjunct Scholar

Laura Jones

Administration

Executive Director, Michael Walker
Director, Finance and Administration, Michael Hopkins
Director, Alberta Policy Research Centre, Barry Cooper
Director, Communications, Suzanne Walters
Director, Development, Sherry Stein
Director, Education Programs, Annabel Addington
Director, Publication Production, J. Kristin McCahon
Events Coordinator, Leah Costello
Coordinator, Student Programs, Vanessa Schneider

Research

Director, Fiscal and Non-Profit Studies, Jason Clemens
Director, School Performance Studies, Peter Cowley
Director, Pharmaceutical Policy Research, John R. Graham
Director, Centre for Studies in Risk, Regulation, and Environment, Kenneth Green
Director, Centre for Trade and Globalization Studies, Fred McMahon
Director, Education Policy, Claudia Rebanks Hepburn
Senior Research Economist, Niels Veldhuis

Ordering publications

To order this book, any other publications, or a catalogue of the Institute's publications, please contact the book sales coordinator via our **toll-free order line: 1.800.665.3558, ext. 580**;
via telephone: 604.688.0221, ext. 580;
via fax: 604.688.8539;
via e-mail: sales@fraserinstitute.ca.

Media

For media information, please contact
Suzanne Walters, Director of Communications:
via telephone: 604.714.4582 or, from Toronto, 416.363.6575, ext. 582;
via e-mail: suzannew@fraserinstitute.ca

Website

To learn more about the Institute and to read our publications on line, please visit our web site at www.fraserinstitute.ca.

Membership

For information about membership, please contact us:

in **Vancouver**,
via mail: The Development Department,
  The Fraser Institute,
  4th Floor, 1770 Burrard Street,
  Vancouver, BC, V6J 3G7;
via telephone: 604.688.0221 ext. 586;
via fax: 604.688.8539;
via e-mail: membership@fraserinstitute.ca;

in **Calgary**,
via telephone: 403.216.7175 or toll-free: 1.866.716.7175;
via fax: 403.234.9010;
via e-mail: barrym@fraserinstitute.ca;

In **Toronto**,
via telephone: 416.363.6575;
via fax: 416.601.7322.

Publication

Editing and design by Kristin McCahon
and Lindsey Thomas Martin

Cover design by Brian Creswick @ GoggleBox.

Risk Controversy Series
General Editor, Laura Jones

The Fraser Institute's Risk Controversy Series publishes a number of short books explaining the science behind today's most pressing public-policy issues, such as global warming, genetic engineering, use of chemicals, and drug approvals. These issues have two common characteristics: they involve complex science and they are controversial, attracting the attention of activists and media. Good policy is based on sound science and sound economics. The purpose of the Risk Controversy Series is to promote good policy by providing Canadians with information from scientists about the complex science involved in many of today's important policy debates. The books in the series are full of valuable information and will provide the interested citizen with a basic understanding of the state of the science, including the many questions that remain unanswered.

Centre for Studies in Risk, Regulation, and Environment

The Fraser Institute's Centre for Studies in Risk, Regulation, and Environment aims to educate Canadian citizens and policy-makers about the science and economics behind risk controversies. As incomes and living standards have increased, tolerance for the risks associated with everyday activities has decreased.

While this decreased tolerance for risk is not undesirable, it has made us susceptible to unsound science. Concern over smaller and smaller risks, both real and imagined, has led us to demand more regulation without taking account of the costs, including foregone opportunities to reduce more threatening risks. If the costs of policies intended to reduce risks are not accounted for, there is a danger that well-intentioned policies will actually reduce public well-being. To promote more rational decision-making, the Centre for Studies in Risk, Regulation, and Environment will focus on sound science and consider the costs as well as the benefits of policies intended to protect Canadians.

For more information about the Centre, contact Kenneth Green, Director, Centre for Studies in Risk, Regulation, and Environment, The Fraser Institute, Fourth Floor, 1770 Burrard Street, Vancouver, BC, V6J 3G7; via telephone: 604.714.4547; via fax: 604.688.8539; via e-mail: keng@fraserinstitute.ca

Misconceptions about the Causes of Cancer

Risk Controversy Series 3

Misconceptions about the Causes of Cancer

Lois Swirsky Gold
Thomas H. Slone
Neela B. Manley
and Bruce N. Ames

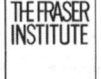 The Fraser Institute
Centre for Studies in Risk, Regulation and Environment
Vancouver British Columbia Canada 2002

Copyright ©2002 by The Fraser Institute. All rights reserved. No part of this book may be reproduced in any manner whatsoever without written permission except in the case of brief passages quoted in critical articles and reviews.

This publication is based on Gold, L. S., Slone, T. H., Ames, B. N., and Manley, N. B. (2001), Pesticide residues in food and cancer risk: A critical analysis, in *Handbook of Pesticide Toxicology* (R. I. Krieger, ed.), Vol. 1, pp. 799–843, Academic Press, New York; and Gold, L. S., Ames, B. N., and Slone, T. H. (2002), Misconceptions about the causes of cancer, in *Human and Environmental Risk Assessment: Theory and Practice* (D. Paustenbach, ed.), pp. 1415–1460, John Wiley & Sons, New York. It was updated and adapted for Canada by the authors.

The authors of this book have worked independently and opinions expressed by them are, therefore, their own and do not necessarily reflect the opinions of the members or the trustees of The Fraser Institute.

Printed in Canada.

National Library of Canada Cataloguing in Publication

Main entry under title:
Misconceptions about the causes of cancer / Lois Swirsky Gold ... [et al.]; general editor, Laura Jones.

   (Risk controversy series ; 3)
   Includes bibliographical references.
   ISBN 0-88975-195-1

   1. Cancer--Environmental aspects.   2. Cancer--Etiology. I. Gold, Lois Swirsky, 1941-   II. Centre for Studies in Risk and Regulation.   III. Series.

RC268.25.M57 2002   616.99'4071   C2002-911284-2

Contents

About the authors / vii

Acknowledgments / ix

Foreword / xi

Summary / 3

Misconception 1—Cancer rates are soaring in the United States and Canada / 5

Misconception 2—Synthetic chemicals at environmental exposure levels are an important cause of human cancer / 7

Misconception 3—Reducing pesticide residues is an effective way to prevent diet-related cancer / 15

Misconception 4—Human exposures to potential cancer hazards are primarily to synthetic chemicals / 23

Misconception 5—The toxicology of synthetic chemicals is different from that of natural chemicals / 27

Misconception 6—Cancer risks to humans can be assessed by standard high-dose animal cancer tests / 31

Misconception 7—Synthetic chemicals pose greater carcinogenic hazards than natural chemicals / 43

Misconception 8—Pesticides and other synthetic chemicals are disrupting hormones / 87

Misconception 9—Regulation of low, hypothetical risks is effective in advancing public health / 89

Glossary / 91

Appendix—Method for calculating the HERP index / 97

References and further reading / 99

About the authors

Lois Swirsky Gold is Director of the Carcinogenic Potency Project and a Senior Scientist, University of California, Berkeley and Lawrence Berkeley National Laboratory. She has published 100 papers on analyses of animal cancer tests and implications for cancer prevention, interspecies extrapolation, and risk assessment methodology. The Carcinogenic Potency Database (CPDB), published as a CRC handbook, analyzes results of 6000 chronic, long-term cancer tests on 1,400 chemicals. Dr. Gold has served on the Panel of Expert Reviewers for the National Toxicology Program, the Boards of the Harvard Center for Risk Analysis, and the Annapolis Center, was a member of the Harvard Risk Management Group and is a member of the Advisory Committee to the Director, National Center for Environmental Health, Centers for Disease Control and Prevention (CDC). She is among the most highly cited scientists in her field and was awarded the Annapolis Center Prize for risk communication. E-mail: cpdb@potency.berkeley.edu

Thomas H. Slone has been a scientist on the Carcinogenic Potency Project at the University of California, Berkeley and at Lawrence Berkeley National Laboratory for 17 years. He has co-authored many of the principal publications of the project. E-mail: cpdb@potency.berkeley.edu

Neela B. Manley has been a scientist on the Carcinogenic Potency Project at the University of California, Berkeley and at Lawrence Berkeley National Laboratory for 13 years. Dr. Manley works on developing the Carcinogenic Potency Database and has co-authored many papers on the project. E-mail: cpdb@potency.berkeley.edu.

Bruce N. Ames is a Professor of Biochemistry and Molecular Biology and is a Senior Scientist at Children's Hospital Oakland Research Institute. He was the Director of the National Institute of Environmental Health Sciences Center, University of California, Berkeley. He is a member of the National Academy of Sciences and was on their Commission on Life Sciences. He was a Member of the National Cancer Advisory Board of the National Cancer Institute (1976–1982). He developed the Ames test for detecting mutagens. Among numerous honors, he is the past recipient of the Japan Prize and the US National Medal of Science. His more than 460 publications have resulted in his being among the few hundred most-cited scientists (all fields). E-mail: BNAmes@UCLink4.Berkeley.edu.

Acknowledgments

We thank the many researchers who have provided data and opinions about their work for development of the Carcinogenic Potency Database, as well as numerous colleagues who have given exposure assessment information for the development of the HERP table and have provided comments on this work over many years. The work of co-authors of earlier papers contributed significantly to this analysis, including particularly Leslie Bernstein, Jerrold Ward, David Freedman, David W. Gaylor, Richard Peto, Margie Profet, and Renae Magaw. We thank Howard Maccabee for reviewing the manuscript. We also thank Kat Wentworth for administrative and technical assistance.

This work was supported by a grant from the Office of Biological and Environmental Research (BER), US Department of Energy, grant number DE-AC03-76SF00098 to L.S.G. at Lawrence Berkeley National Laboratory; by the National Institute of Environmental Health Sciences Center Grant ESO1896 at the University of California, Berkeley; and by a grant for research in disease prevention through the Dean's Office of the College of Letters and Science, University of California, Berkeley to LSG and BNA.

Foreword

Misconceptions about the Causes of Cancer is the third publication in The Centre for Studies in Risk and Regulation's Risk Controversy Series, which will explain the science behind many of today's most pressing public-policy issues. Many current public-policy issues such as global warming, genetic engineering, use of chemicals, and drug approvals have two common characteristics: they involve complex science and they are controversial, attracting the attention of environmental activists and media. The mix of complex science, alarmist hype, and short media clips can bewilder the concerned citizen.

The environmental alarmists

The development and use of new technology has long attracted an "anti" movement. Recent high-profile campaigns include those against globalization, genetic engineering, cell phones, breast implants, greenhouse gases, and plastic softeners used in children's toys. To convince people that the risks from these products or technologies warrant attention, alarmists rely on dramatic pictures, public protests, and slogans to attract media attention and capture the public's imagination. The goal of these campaigns is not to educate people so they can make informed choices for themselves—the goal is to regulate or, preferably, to eliminate the offending product or technology. While the personal motivations of alarmists vary, their campaigns have three common characteristics. First, there is an underlying suspicion of economic development. Many prominent environmentalists, for example, say that economic growth is the enemy of the environment and among anti-globalization crusaders, "multinational corporation" is a dirty word. Second, the benefits of the products, technologies, or life-styles that are attacked are ignored while the risks are emphasized and often exaggerated. Some anti-technology groups will insist that a product or technology be proven to pose no risk at all before it is brought to market—this is sometimes called the precautionary principle. This may sound sensible but it is, in fact, an absurd demand: nothing, including many products that we use and activities we enjoy daily, is completely safe. Even the simple act of eating an apple poses some risk—one could choke on the apple or the apple might damage a tooth. Finally, environmental activist groups have a tendency to focus only on arguments that support their claims, while often dismissing legitimate scientific debates and ignoring uncertainty: they claim, for example, that there is a consensus among scientists that global warming is caused largely by human activity and that something must therefore be done to control greenhouse gas emissions. As the first publication in this series showed, no such consensus exists.

The media

Many of us rely exclusively on the media for information on topics of current interest as, understandably, we do not have time to conduct our own, more thorough literature reviews and investigations. For business and political news as well as for human-interest stories, newspaper, radio, and television media do a good job of keeping us informed. But, these topics are relatively straight-forward to cover as they involve familiar people, terms, and places. Stories involving complex science are harder to do. Journalists covering these stories often do not have a scientific background and, even with a scientific background, it is difficult to condense and simplify scientific issues for viewers or readers. Finally, journalists work on tight deadlines, often having less than a day to research and write a story. Tight deadlines also make it tempting to rely on activists who are eager to provide information and colorful quotations.

Relying on media for information about a complex scientific issue can also give one an unbalanced view of the question because bad news is a better story than good news. In his book, *A Moment on the Earth*, Gregg Easterbrook, a reporter who has covered environmental issues for *Newsweek*, *The New Republic*, and *The New York Times Magazine*, explains the asymmetry in the way the media cover environmental stories.

> In the autumn of 1992, I was struck by this headline in the *New York Times*: "Air Found Cleaner in US Cities." The accompanying story said that in the past five years air quality had improved sufficiently that nearly half the cities once violating federal smog standards no longer did so. I was also struck by how the *Times* treated the article—as a small box buried on page A24. I checked the nation's other important news organizations and learned that none had given the finding prominence. Surely any news that air quality was in decline would have received front-page attention (p. xiii).

Despite dramatic overall improvements in air quality in Canada over the past 30 years, stories about air quality in Canada also focus on the bad news. Both the *Globe and Mail* and the *National Post* emphasized reports that air quality was deteriorating. Eighty-nine percent of the *Globe and Mail*'s coverage of air quality and 81 percent of the *National Post*'s stories in 2000 focused on poor air quality (Miljan,

Air Quality Improving—But You'd Never Know It from the *Globe & Post*, *Fraser Forum*, April 2001: 17–18).

That bad news makes a better story than good news is a more generally observable phenomenon. According to the Pew Research Center for the People and the Press, each of the top 10 stories of public interest in the United States during 1999 were about bad news. With the exception of the outcome of the American election, the birth of septuplets in Iowa, and the summer Olympics, the same is true for the top 10 stories in each year from 1996 through 1998 (Pew Research Center for the People and the Press 2000, digital document: www.people-press.org/yearendrpt.htm).

While it is tempting to blame the media for over-simplifying complicated scientific ideas and presenting only the bad news, we must remember that they are catering to the desires of their readers and viewers. Most of us rely on newspapers, radio, and television because we want simple, interesting stories. We also find bad news more interesting than good news. Who would buy a paper that had "Millions of Airplanes land safely in Canada each Year" as its headline? But, many of us are drawn to headlines that promise a story giving gory details of a plane crash.

The Risk Controversy Series

Good policy is based on sound science and sound economics. The purpose of the Risk Controversy Series is to promote good policy by providing Canadians with information from scientists about the complex science involved in many of today's important policy debates. While these reports are not as short or as easy to read as a news story, they are full of valuable information and will provide the interested citizen with a basic understanding of the state of the science, including the many questions that remain unanswered.

Laura Jones, Adjunct Scholar
The Fraser Institute

Misconceptions about the causes of cancer

Summary

The major avoidable causes of cancer are: (1) smoking, which accounts for 27% of cancer deaths in Canada and 80% to 90% of deaths from lung cancer; (2) dietary imbalances (e.g., lack of sufficient amounts of dietary fruits and vegetables), which account for about another third; (3) chronic infections, mostly in developing countries; and (4) hormonal factors, which are influenced primarily by life-style.

There is no cancer epidemic except for lung cancer due to smoking. (Cancer is actually many diseases, and the causes differ for cancers at different target sites.) Since 1971, overall cancer mortality rates in Canada (excluding lung cancer) have declined 17% in women and 5% in men. Regulatory policy that focuses on traces of synthetic chemicals is based on misconceptions about animal cancer tests. Current research indicates that it is not rare for substances to cause cancer in laboratory rodents in the standard high-dose experiments. Half of all chemicals tested, whether occurring naturally or produced synthetically, are "carcinogens"; there are high-dose effects in rodent cancer tests that are not relevant to low-dose human exposures and which may contribute to the high proportion of chemicals that test positive.

The focus of regulatory policy is on synthetic chemicals, but 99.9% of the chemicals humans ingest are natural.

For example, more than 1000 naturally occurring chemicals have been described in coffee: 30 have been tested and 21 have been found to be carcinogenic in rodents in high-dose tests. Plants in the human diet contain thousands of natural "pesticides" produced by plants to protect themselves from insects and other predators: 72 have been tested and 38 have been found to give cancer to rodents. Thus, exposure to synthetic rodent carcinogens is small compared to the natural background of rodent carcinogens. High-dose rodent cancer tests need to be re-evaluated by viewing results from this perspective.

There is no convincing evidence that synthetic chemical pollutants are important as a cause of human cancer. Regulations targeted to eliminate low levels of synthetic chemicals are enormously expensive: the United States Environmental Protection Agency (EPA) has estimated that environmental regulations cost $140 billion per year in the United States. Others have estimated that the median toxic control program costs 146 times more per hypothetical life-year saved than the median medical intervention. Attempting to reduce low hypothetical risks has other costs as well: if reducing synthetic pesticides makes fruits and vegetables more expensive, thereby decreasing consumption, then the cancer rate will likely increase. The prevention of cancer will come from knowledge obtained from biomedical research, education of the public, and life-style changes made by individuals. A re-examination of priorities in cancer prevention, both public and private, seems called for.

In this study, we highlight nine misconceptions about pollution, pesticides, and the causes of cancer. We briefly present the scientific evidence that undermines each misconception. The nine misconceptions are listed in **Contents** (p. v–vi) and an extensive bibliography is provided in **References and further reading** (p. 99). Phrases in the text typeset like this, *carcinogenic potency*, are defined in the **Glossary** (p. 91).

Misconception 1—Cancer rates are soaring in the United States and Canada

Overall cancer death rates in Canada (excluding lung cancer due to smoking) have declined 17% in women and 5% in men since 1971 (National Cancer Institute of Canada 2001). In the United States, the decline is similar: overall cancer death rates (excluding lung cancer) have declined 19% since 1950 (Ries & al. 2000).

In Canada, the types of cancer deaths that have decreased since 1971 are primarily stomach, cervical, and colorectal (National Cancer Institute of Canada 2001). Those that have increased are primarily lung cancer (80%–90% is due to smoking in Canada (American Cancer Society 2000; Manuel & Hockin 2000)), melanoma (probably due to sunburns), and non-Hodgkin's lymphoma (National Cancer Institute of Canada 2001). If lung cancer is included, current cancer mortality rates (Ries & al. 2000) are similar to those in 1972 (National Cancer Institute of Canada 2001). For some cancers, mortality rates have begun to decline due in part to early detection, treatment, and improved survival (American Cancer Society 2000; Linet & al. 1999), as is the case with breast cancer in women (National Cancer Institute of Canada 2001; Peto & al. 2000). The rise in incidence rates in older age groups for some cancers can be explained by known factors such as improved screening (Bailar & Gornik 1997; Devesa & al. 1995; Doll & Peto 1981; Peto & al. 2000): "The reason for not focusing on the reported incidence of cancer is that the scope and precision of diagnostic information, practices in screening and early detection, and criteria for reporting cancer have changed so much over time that trends in incidence are not reliable" (Bailar & Gornik 1997: 1569–70). Changes in incidence rates are thus complicated to interpret. For some cancers, in addition to earlier screening and diagnosis, increases in incidence over time are known to be associated with lifestyle factors; e.g. for breast cancer, having fewer children and having them later in life.

Life expectancy has continued to rise since 1921 (Anderson 1999; Manuel & Hockin 2000): in Canada, life expectancy in the early 1920s was 59 years (http://www.statcan.ca/english/Pgdb/People/Health/health26.htm); today it is about 79 years (World Health Organization 1984). Trends in the United States are similar to those in Canada (Anderson 1999).

Misconception 2—Synthetic chemicals at environmental exposure levels are an important cause of human cancer

Studies of cancer rates around the world indicate that the major avoidable causes of cancer primarily reflect lifestyle or other environmental factors that can be modified to reduce cancer risk (i.e. factors that are not genetic) (Armstrong & Doll 1975; Doll & Peto 1981). The main evidence for this conclusion is that rates of cancer in specific organs differ markedly in different countries; when people migrate to other countries their cancer rates change and within a few generations usually resemble the rates in their new countries. Additionally, rates change over time in a given country.

Neither *epidemiology* nor toxicology supports the idea that exposures to synthetic industrial chemicals at the levels at which they are generally found in the environment are important as a cause of human cancer (Ames & al. 1995; Devesa & al. 1995; Gold & al. 1992).

Instead, other environmental factors have been identified in epidemiological studies that are likely to have a major effect on lowering cancer rates: reduction of smoking, improving diet (e.g. increased consumption of fruits and vegetables), hormonal factors (some of which are diet-related), and control of infections (Ames & al. 1995).

Few epidemiological studies find an association between the risk of cancer and low levels of industrial pollutants or pesticide residues; the associations are usually weak, the results are often conflicting, and the studies usually do not address individual pesticides (Dich & al. 1997). Moreover, the studies often do not correct for potentially large *confounding factors* such as composition of the diet (Ames 1998; Ames & al. 1995; Doll & Peto 1981; Gold & al. 2001a, http://monographs.iarc.fr/monoeval/crthgr01.html; International Agency for Research on Cancer 1971–2001). Epidemiological studies on the risk of breast cancer have found no association with pesticide residues (Gammon & al. 2002; Grodstein & al. 1997; Hunter & al. 1998). The most recent *case-control study* measured residues in blood of DDT, DDE, dieldrin, and chlordane and found no association with breast cancer (Gammon & al. 2002).

From the toxicological perspective, exposures to synthetic pollutants are at very low levels and, therefore, rarely seem plausible as a causal factor, particularly when compared to the background of natural chemicals in the diet that are carcinogenic in rodents in high-dose tests (i.e. rodent carcinogens) (Ames & al. 1990a; Gold & al. 1997b; Gold & al. 1992). Even if one assumes that the worst-case risk estimates for synthetic pollutants are true risks, the proportion of cancer that the United States Environmental Protection Agency (EPA) could prevent by regulation would be tiny (Gough 1990). Historically, some high occupational exposures to some industrial chemicals have caused human cancer, though estimating the proportion of all cancers that are due to occupational exposures has been a controversial issue: a few percent seems a reasonable estimate (Ames & al. 1995; Doll & Peto 1981), and much of this is from asbestos in smokers. Exposures to synthetic chemicals or industrial mixtures in the workplace can be much higher than the exposure to chemicals in food, air, or water. Past occupational exposures have sometimes been high, and about half the agents that have been evaluated as human carcinogens by International Agency for Research on Cancer (IARC) were identified by workplace exposures. Since occupational cancer is concentrated among small groups with high levels of exposure, there is an opportunity to control or eliminate risks once they are identified. In the United States, Permissible Exposure Limits in the workplace are sometimes close to the carcinogenic dose in rodents (Gold & al. 1994a) and, thus, require priority attention. See **Misconception 7** (p. 43).

Aging and cancer

Cancer is due, in part, to normal aging and increases exponentially with age in both rodents and humans (Ames & al. 1993b). To the extent that the major avoidable risk factors for cancer are diminished, cancer will occur at later ages and the proportion of cancer caused by normal metabolic processes will increase. Aging and its degenerative diseases appear to be due in part to *oxidative damage* to DNA and other macromolecules (Ames & al. 1993b; Beckman & Ames 1998). By-products of normal metabolism—superoxide, hydrogen peroxide, and hydroxyl radical—are the same *oxidative mutagens* produced by radiation. *Mitochondria* from old animals leak oxidants (Hagen & al. 1997): old rats have been estimated to have about 66,000 *oxidative DNA lesions* per cell (Helbock & al. 1998), although methods to measure such lesions are improving and may change the number somewhat. DNA is oxidized in normal metabolism because antioxidant defenses, though numerous, are not perfect. Antioxidant defenses against oxidative damage include vitamin C (Rice-Evans & al. 1997) which comes from dietary fruits and vegetables, and vitamin E (Rice-Evans & al. 1997), which comes from nuts, vegetable oils, and fat. In addition, mitochondria, the organelles in the cell that generate energy and are the main source of oxidants, may need different antioxidants (Hagen & al. 2002; Liu & al. 2002a; Liu

& al. 2002b). Increasing antioxidant intake in those persons with low intakes may help to prevent cancer but it is difficult to disentangle dietary intake of individual vitamins or minerals in epidemiological studies (Ames & Wakimoto 2002).

Smoking

In Canada, smoking contributes to 27% of cancer deaths and about 45,000 premature deaths per year (American Cancer Society 2000; Makomaski Illing & Kaiserman 1999; National Cancer Institute of Canada 2000; Ries & al. 2000). Overall, 21% of deaths from the three leading causes of death (cancer, heart disease, and cerebrovascular disease) are attributable to smoking (Makomaski Illing & Kaiserman 1999). Tobacco is a cause of cancer of the lung, mouth, pharynx, larynx, esophagus, bladder, pancreas, stomach, kidney, uterine cervix, and myeloid leukemia (International Agency for Research on Cancer 1986; International Agency for Research on Cancer 2002, in press). Smoke contains a wide variety of mutagens and substances that are carcinogenic in rodents. Smoking is also a severe *oxidative stress* and causes inflammation in the lung. The oxidants in cigarette smoke—mainly nitrogen oxides—deplete the body's antioxidants (Lykkesfeldt & al. 2000). Thus, smokers need to ingest more vitamin C than non-smokers to achieve the same level in blood but they tend not to do so: an inadequate concentration of vitamin C in plasma is more common among smokers (Lykkesfeldt & al. 2000). A recent Danish study indicated that smokers consumed fewer fruits and vegetables than nonsmokers (Osler & al. 2002). Additionally, people who take supplements of vitamins and minerals are less likely to be smokers (Patterson & al. 2001).

Men with inadequate diets or who smoke may damage the DNA in all cells of the body, including their sperm. When the level of dietary vitamin C is insufficient to keep vitamin C in the seminal fluid at an adequate level, the oxidative lesions in sperm DNA are increased 2.5 times (Ames

& al. 1994; Fraga & al. 1991; Fraga & al. 1996). Male smokers have more oxidative lesions in sperm DNA (Fraga & al. 1996) and more chromosomal abnormalities in sperm (Wyrobek & al. 1995) than do nonsmokers. It is plausible, therefore, that fathers who smoke may increase the risk of birth defects and childhood cancer in offspring (Ames & al. 1994; Fraga & al. 1991; Woodall & Ames 1997). Some epidemiological studies suggest that the rate of childhood cancers is increased in offspring of male smokers (Ji & al. 1997; Sorahan & al. 1995).

Involuntary (environmental) exposure to tobacco smoke (i.e. "second-hand smoke") has also been evaluated as a human carcinogen (International Agency for Research on Cancer 2002, in press; US Department of Heath and Human Services 1986; US Environmental Protection Agency 1992b), and is estimated to increase the risk of lung cancer by 20% to 30%. In comparison, smokers have an increased risk of lung cancer of 2000% (International Agency for Research on Cancer 2002, in press), i.e. 600 to 1000 times greater risk than from involuntary smoking.

Diet

Dietary factors have been estimated to account for about one third of cancer deaths in the United States (American Cancer Society 2000; Ames & al. 1995; Doll & Peto 1981; Ries & al. 2000) and specific dietary factors are slowly being clarified, although epidemiological research on diet has many complexities and confounding factors. Low intake of fruits and vegetables is associated with increased cancer incidence in many case-control studies (Block & al. 1992; World Cancer Research Fund 1997); results from several recent *cohort studies*, however, have been less consistent (Willett 2001). (See **Misconception 3**, p. 15). Excessive consumption of alcoholic beverages is associated with cancers of the breast, oral cavity (primarily in smokers), and liver (International Agency for Research on Cancer 1988; Willett 2001).

There has been considerable interest in calories (and dietary fat) as a risk factor for cancer, in part because caloric restriction markedly lowers the cancer rate and increases life span in rodents (Ames & al. 1995; Hart & al. 1995b; Turturro & al. 1996; Vainio & Bianchini 2002). For two common cancers, breast and colon, international comparisons in incidence suggested a role for fat intake; however, combined analyses of many studies do not support such an association (Hunter & al. 1996; Willett 2001). Higher intake of dietary fiber does not appear to protect against colon cancer, although some earlier case-control studies suggested that it did (Willett 2001). Current scientific attention has focused on body weight (obesity), weight gain among adults, and inadequate physical activity as risk factors for cancer (Caan & al. 1998; Giovannucci & al. 1995; Huang & al. 1997; Vainio & Bianchini 2002; Willett 2001). A recent report by IARC states:

> Taken together, excess body weight and physical inactivity account for approximately one fourth to one third of breast cancer, cancers of the colon, endometrium, kidney (renal cell) and oesophagus (adenocarcinoma). Thus adiposity and inactivity appear to be the most important avoidable causes of postmenopausal breast cancer, endometrial cancer, renal cell cancer, and adenocarcinoma of the oesophagus, and among the most important avoidable causes of colon cancer. (Vainio & Bianchini 2002)

Lack of regular physical activity contributes independently to risk of colon (Giovannucci & al. 1995; Giovannucci & al. 1996; Martinez & al. 1997; Platz & al. 2000; Willett 2001) and breast cancer (Bernstein & al. 1994; Rockhill & al. 1999; Willett 2001).

Hormonal factors
Endogenous reproductive hormones play a large role in cancer, including that of the breast, prostate, ovary, and

endometrium (Henderson & Feigelson 2000; Henderson & al. 1991), contributing to about 20% of all cancer. Many life-style factors such as reproductive history, lack of exercise, obesity, and intake of alcohol influence hormone levels and therefore affect risk (Ames & al. 1995; Henderson & Feigelson 2000; Henderson & al. 1991; Hunter & Willett 1993; Kelsey & Bernstein 1996; Writing Group for the Women's Health Initiative Investigators 2002). The mechanisms for postmenopausal breast cancer may involve changes in hormone metabolism: e.g. earlier menstruation and postmenopausal release of estrogen from body fat, never having a child, giving birth for the first time over age 35, or hormone replacement therapy. Recent results of a clinical trial in the study by the Women's Health Initiative indicate that hormone-replacement therapy (estrogen and progestin) increases the risk of postmenopausal breast cancer (Writing Group for the Women's Health Initiative Investigators 2002).

Chronic inflammation
Chronic inflammation results in the release of oxidative mutagens from white cells and other sentinel cells of the immune system, which combat bacteria, parasites, and viruses by destroying them with potent, mutagenic oxidizing agents (Ames & al. 1995; Christen & al. 1999). These oxidants protect humans from immediate death from infection but they also cause oxidative damage to DNA, chronic killing of cells with compensatory cell division, and mutation (Shacter & al. 1988; Yamashina & al. 1986); thus, they contribute to cancer. Anti-inflammatory agents, including some antioxidants, appear to inhibit some of the pathology of chronic inflammation. Chronic infections such as hepatitis B and C, viruses and liver cancer, *Helicobacter pylori* and stomach cancer that give rise to chronic inflammation are estimated to cause about 21% of new cancer cases in developing countries and 9% in developed countries (Pisani &

al. 1997). Obesity is associated with a systemic chronic inflammation, which suggests that it may play a role in cancer risk (Das 2001).

Other factors

Other causal factors in human cancer are excessive exposure to the sun, viruses (e.g., human papillomavirus and cervical cancer), and pharmaceuticals (e.g. phenacetin, some chemotherapy agents, diethylstilbestrol, estrogens). Genetic factors affect susceptibility to cancer and interact with life-style and other risk factors. Biomedical research is uncovering important genetic variation in humans that can affect susceptibility.

Misconception 3—Reducing pesticide residues is an effective way to prevent diet-related cancer

Reduction in the use of pesticides will not effectively prevent diet-related cancer. Diets high in fruits and vegetables, which are the source of most human exposures to pesticide residues, are associated with reduced risk of many types of cancer. Less use of synthetic pesticides would increase costs of fruits and vegetables and, thus, likely reduce consumption, especially among people with low incomes, who spend a higher percentage of their income on food.

Dietary fruits and vegetables and cancer prevention

Two types of evidence, (1) *epidemiological* studies on diet and cancer and (2) laboratory studies on vitamin or mineral inadequacy, support the idea that low intake of fruits and vegetables is associated with increased risk of degenerative diseases, including cancer, cardiovascular disease, cataracts, and brain dysfunction (Ames & al. 1995; Ames & al. 1993b; Ames & Wakimoto 2002). Fruits and vegetables are an important source of essential vitamins and minerals (Ames & Wakimoto 2002).

Despite the evidence about the importance of fruits and vegetables, the Canadian campaign "5-to-10-a-Day:

Are You Getting Enough?" reported that 67% of Canadians do not eat 5 or more servings of fruits and vegetables per day, based on a Nielson telephone survey of women (http://5to10aday.com/eng/media_news_nr1.htm; A. Matyas, pers. comm.). Another survey, by interview, reported that about half of Canadians do not eat 5 servings or more per day (Gray-Donald & al. 2000). In the United States, it has been estimated that 80% of children and adolescents, and 68% of adults (Krebs-Smith & al. 1995; Krebs-Smith & al. 1996) do not eat 5 servings or more per day. Publicity about hundreds of minor, hypothetical risks, such as pesticide residues, can result in a loss of perspective on what is important (US National Cancer Institute 1996): only 7% of Canadians surveyed thought that eating fruits and vegetables can reduce the risk of cancer (http://www.5to10aday.com/eng/media_executive_summary.htm). There is a paradox in the public concern about possible cancer hazards from the low levels of pesticide residues in food and the lack of public understanding of the evidence that eating *more* of the main foods that contain pesticide residues—fruits and vegetables—protects against cancer.

Several reviews of the epidemiological literature show that a high proportion of **case-control studies** find an inverse association between fruit and vegetable consumption and cancer risk (Block & al. 1992; Hill & al. 1994; Steinmetz & Potter 1996; World Cancer Research Fund 1997). It is not clear from these studies whether individuals who consume very low amounts are the only people at risk, that is, whether there is an adequate level above which there is no increased cancer risk. Table 1 reports the number and proportion of case-control studies for each type of cancer, that show a statistically significant protective effect (World Cancer Research Fund 1997). A recent international panel considered the evidence of a protective effect of fruits and vegetables most convincing for cancers of the oral cav-

Table 1: Review of epidemiological (case-control) studies worldwide on the association between cancer risk and the consumption of fruit and vegetables

Cancer site	Proportion of studies with statistically significant protective effect of fruits and/or vegetables*	Percent of studies with protective effect
Larynx	6/6	100%
Stomach	28/30	93%
Mouth, oral cavity, & pharynx	13/15	87%
Bladder	6/7	86%
Lung	11/13	85%
Esophagus	15/18	83%
Pancreas	9/11	82%
Cervix	4/5	80%
Endometrium	4/5	80%
Rectum	8/10	80%
Colon	15/19	79%
Colon/rectum	3/5	60%
Breast	8/12	67%
Thyroid	3/5	60%
Kidney	3/5	60%
Prostate	1/6	17%
Nasal & nasopharynx	2/4	—
Ovary	3/4	—
Skin	2/2	—
Vulva	1/1	—
Mesothelium	0/1	—
Total	144/183	79%

Source: World Cancer Research Fund 1997.
Note *: p<0.05 for test for trend, p<0.05 for odds ratio for uppermost consumption level, or 95% confidence interval excluding 1.0 for uppermost consumption level.
Note: "—" = fewer than 5 studies, so no percent was calculated.

ity, esophagus, stomach, and lung (World Cancer Research Fund 1997). In another review, the median relative risk was about 2 for the quarter of the population with the lowest dietary intake of fruits and vegetables compared to the quarter with the highest intake for cancers of the lung, larynx, oral cavity, esophagus, stomach, bladder, pancreas, and cervix (Block & al. 1992). The median relative risk was not as high for the hormonally related cancers of breast, prostate, and ovary, or for the colon.

More than 30 large cohort studies of the relationship between diet and cancer are in progress in various countries (Willett 2001). Generally the results of *cohort studies* have been less strong and less consistent than case-control studies in their findings about the association between fruit and vegetable intake and cancer risk (Botterweck & al. 1998; Galanis & al. 1998; Giovannucci & al. 2002; Jansen & al. 2001; Kasum & al. 2002; McCullough & al. 2001; Michels & al. 2000; Ozasa & al. 2001; Schuurman & al. 1998; Sellers & al. 1998; Smith-Warner & al. 2001; Terry & al. 1998; Terry & al. 2001; Voorrips & al. 2000; Zeegers & al. 2001). Some cohort studies have shown a lack of association between fruit and vegetable consumption and cancers of the colon, breast, and stomach (Botterweck & al. 1998; Galanis & al. 1998; Kasum & al. 2002; McCullough & al. 2001; Michels & al. 2000; Sellers & al. 1998; Smith-Warner & al. 2001; Terry & al. 1998; Terry & al. 2001; Voorrips & al. 2000). As more analyses are reported from cohort studies, the estimation of relative risks should become more precise.

Observational epidemiological studies have many limitations that make interpretation of results complex. Unlike experiments in rodents, in which a single variable is changed and everything else is controlled for, in epidemiological studies on diet, people eat varied diets and change over time, they may not recall correctly their eating habits, and they have different genetic makeups. Some examples of the kinds of complexities in these studies follow.

The category "fruits and vegetables" is broad and foods contain different amounts of each vitamin or mineral. If a minimum amount of a specific vitamin or mineral is required for protection against a specific cancer, then it may be inadequacy of individual foods that is related to risk (Willett 2001). This is usually not the focus in research investigations; rather, the focus is the combined category, fruits and vegetables. Additionally, use of a multivitamin pill or of a particular vitamin pill has generally not been taken into account in these studies and this may *confound* the results because those who take supplements have a healthier lifestyle that includes a greater intake of fruits and vegetables as well as other factors like lower rates of smoking, diets lower in fat, and a belief in the connection between diet and cancer that may affect both their behaviors and their recall of dietary intakes (Block & al. 1994; Patterson & al. 2001). Methodological limitations of case-control studies that may account for findings that are stronger than those of cohort studies include *recall bias*—controls may remember their dietary habits differently from cases (the people with cancer)—and selection bias—people who choose to participate as controls may have healthier life-styles that include, among other factors, a higher intake of fruits and vegetables, which leads, in turn, to a lower observed relative risk that may not really be due to fruits and vegetables.

Inadequate intake of vitamins and minerals

Laboratory studies of vitamin and mineral inadequacy indicate an association with DNA damage, which suggests that the vitamin and mineral content of fruits and vegetables may underlie the observed association between the intake of fruits and vegetables and the risk of cancer. Maximum health and lifespan require metabolic harmony; and inadequate or sub-optimal intake of essential vitamins and minerals may result in metabolic damage that can affect many functions and hence affect the development of diseases.

Antioxidants such as vitamin C (whose dietary source is fruits and vegetables), vitamin E, and selenium protect against *oxidative damage* caused by normal metabolism (Helbock & al. 1998), smoking (Ames 1998), and inflammation (Ames & al. 1993b) (See **Misconception #2**). *Deficiency* of some vitamins and minerals can mimic radiation in damaging DNA by causing single- and double-strand breaks, or oxidative lesions, or both (Ames 1998). Those vitamins and minerals whose deficiency appears to mimic radiation are folic acid, B_{12}, B_6, niacin, C, E, iron, and zinc, with the laboratory evidence ranging from likely to compelling. In the United States, the percentage of the population that consumes less than half the recommmended daily allowance (RDA) in the diet (i.e. ignoring supplement use) for five of these eight vitamins or minerals is estimated to be: zinc—10% of women/men older than 50; iron—25% of menstruating women and 5% of women over 50; vitamin C—25% of women/men; folate—50% of women and 25% of men; vitamin B—10% of women/men; vitamin B_{12}—10% of women and 5% of men (Ames & Wakimoto 2002). A considerable percentage of the United States population may be deficient in some vitamin or mineral (Ames 1998; Ames & Wakimoto 2002).

A deficiency of folic acid, one of the most common vitamin deficiencies in the population consuming few dietary fruits and vegetables, causes chromosome breaks in humans (Blount & al. 1997). The mechanism of chromosome breaks has been shown to be analogous to radiation (Blount & al. 1997). Folate supplementation above the RDA minimized chromosome breakage (Fenech & al. 1998). Folate deficiency has been associated with increased risk of colon cancer (Giovannucci & al. 1993; Mason 1994): in the Nurses' Health Study women who took a multivitamin supplement containing folate for 15 years had a 75% lower risk of colon cancer (Giovannucci & al. 1998). Folate deficiency also damages human sperm (Wallock & al. 2001), causes neural tube defects in the fetus, and an estimated 10% of heart disease in the United States (Boushey & al. 1995). Approximately 10% of the American population (Senti & Pilch 1985) had a lower folate level than that at which chromosome breaks occur (Blount & al. 1997). Nearly 20 years ago, two small studies of low-income (mainly African-American) elderly (Bailey & al. 1979) and adolescents (Bailey & al. 1982) showed that about half the people in both groups studied had folate levels that low. Recently in Canada and the United States, flour, rice, pasta, and cornmeal have been supplemented with folate (Health Canada 1998; Jacques & al. 1999).

Recent evidence indicates that a deficiency of vitamin B_6 works by the same mechanism as folate deficiency and this would cause chromosome breaks (Huang, Shultz & Ames, unpublished). Niacin contributes to the repair of DNA strand-breaks by maintaining nicotinamide adenine dinucleotide levels for the poly ADP-ribose protective response to DNA damage (Zhang & al. 1993). As a result, dietary insufficiencies of niacin (15% of some populations are deficient) (Jacobson 1993), folate, and antioxidants may interact synergistically to affect the synthesis and repair of DNA adversely. Diets deficient in fruits and vegetables are commonly low in folate, antioxidants, (e.g., vitamin C), and many other vitamins and minerals, result in DNA damage, and are associated with higher cancer rates (Ames 1998; Ames & al. 1995; Block & al. 1992; Subar & al. 1989).

Vitamins and minerals from dietary sources other than fruits and vegetables

Vitamins and minerals whose main dietary sources are other than fruits and vegetables, are also likely to play a significant role in the prevention and repair of DNA damage, and thus are important to the maintenance of long-term health (Ames 1998). Deficiency of vitamin B_{12} (whose source in animal products) causes a functional folate deficiency, accumulation of homocysteine (a risk factor for heart disease) (Herbert & Filer 1996), and chromosome breaks. B_{12} supplementation above the RDA was necessary to minimize chromosome breakage (Fenech & al. 1998). Strict vegetarians are at increased risk for developing vitamin B_{12} deficiency (Herbert & Filer 1996).

Epidemiological studies of supplement usage (vitamin and mineral intake by pill) have shown at most only modest support for an association. The strongest protective effect was for vitamin E and cancers of the prostate and colon (Patterson & al. 2001). There are many potential problems in conducting such studies including the need and difficulty in measuring supplement use over a long period of time, potential confounding of supplement usage with many other aspects of a healthy life-style, such as more exercise, better diet, and not smoking (Patterson & al. 2001). Clinical trials of supplements are generally too short to measure cancer risk since cancers usually develop slowly and the risk increases with age; moreover, such trials cannot measure the potential reduction in risk if supplements are taken throughout a lifetime (Block 1995). Additionally, the cancer risks of supplement users may be overestimated because they are more likely to undergo early screening like mammograms or tests for prostate cancer (prostate-specific antigen, PSA) which are associated with increased diagnosis (Patterson & al. 2001). Such confounding factors are not measured in many epidemiological studies.

Intake of adequate amounts of vitamins and minerals may have a major effect on health, and the costs and risks of a daily multivitamin and mineral pill are low (Ames 1998). More research in this area, as well as efforts to improve diets, should be high priorities for public policy.

Misconception 4—Human exposures to potential cancer hazards are primarily to synthetic chemicals

Contrary to common perception, 99.9% of the chemicals humans ingest are natural. The amounts of synthetic pesticide residues in plant foods, for example, are extremely low compared to the amounts of natural "pesticides" produced by plants themselves (Ames & al. 1990a; Ames & al. 1990b; Gold & al. 1999; Gold & al. 1997b; Gold & Zeiger 1997). Of all dietary pesticides that humans eat, 99.99% are natural: these are chemicals produced by plants to defend themselves against fungi, insects, and other animal predators (Ames & al. 1990a; Ames & al. 1990b). Each plant produces a different array of such chemicals. On average, the Western diet includes roughly 5,000 to 10,000 different natural pesticides and their break-down products. Americans eat about 1,500 mg of natural pesticides per person per day, which is about 10,000 times more than they consume of synthetic pesticide residues (Ames & al. 1990b). Even though only a small proportion of natural pesticides has been tested for carcinogenicity, half of those tested (38/72) have been found to be carcinogenic in rodents; naturally occurring pesticides that are rodent carcinogens are ubiquitous in fruits, vegetables, herbs, and spices (Gold & al. 1997b; Gold & al. 1992) (table 2). Cooking of foods produces burnt material—about 2,000 mg per person per day—that also contains many rodent carcinogens.

In contrast, the residues of 200 synthetic chemicals measured by United States Federal Drug Administration, including the synthetic pesticides thought to be of greatest importance, average only about 0.09 mg per person per day (Ames & al. 1990a; Gold & al. 1997b; Gold & al. 1992). In a single cup of coffee, the natural chemicals that are rodent carcinogens are about equal in weight to an entire year's worth of synthetic pesticide residues that are rodent carcinogens, even though only 3% of the natural chemicals in roasted coffee have been adequately tested for carcinogenicity (Gold & al. 1992) (table 3). This does not mean that coffee or natural pesticides are a cancer risk for humans, but rather that assumptions about high-dose animal cancer tests for assessing human risk at low doses need reexamination. No diet can be free of natural chemicals that are rodent carcinogens (Gold & al. 1999; Gold & al. 1997b; Gold & Zeiger 1997).

The emphasis in cancer bioassays of testing synthetic chemicals means that only minimal data are available on the enormous background of naturally occurring chemicals. If many of the natural chemicals were tested, it is likely that many dietary constituents would be carcinogens in high-dose animal tests. The importance for human cancer of any single rodent carcinogen in the diet is questionable because of the ubiquitous occurrence of so many naturally occurring chemicals that have not been tested and the fact that half of those tested are positive in such tests (**Misconception 6, p. 31**).

Misconceptions about the Causes of Cancer

Table 2. Carcinogenicity status of natural pesticides tested in rodents[a]

Carcinogens: $N = 38$	acetaldehyde methylformylhydrazone, allyl isothiocyanate, arecoline.HCl, benzaldehyde, benzyl acetate, caffeic acid, capsaicin, catechol, clivorine, coumarin, crotonaldehyde, 3,4-dihydrocoumarin, estragole, ethyl acrylate, $N2$-γ-glutamyl-p-hydrazinobenzoic acid, hexanal methylformylhydrazine, p-hydrazinobenzoic acid.HCl, hydroquinone, 1-hydroxyanthraquinone, lasiocarpine, d-limonene, 3-methoxycatechol, 8-methoxypsoralen, N-methyl-N-formylhydrazine, α-methylbenzyl alcohol, 3-methylbutanal methylformylhydrazone, 4-methylcatechol, methyl eugenol, methylhydrazine, monocrotaline, pentanal methylformylhydrazone, petasitenine, quercetin, reserpine, safrole, senkirkine, sesamol, symphytine
Noncarcinogens: $N = 34$	atropine, benzyl alcohol, benzyl isothiocyanate, benzyl thiocyanate, biphenyl, d-carvone, codeine, deserpidine, disodium glycyrrhizinate, ephedrine sulphate, epigallocatechin, eucalyptol, eugenol, gallic acid, geranyl acetate, β-N-[γ-l(+)-glutamyl]-4-hydroxymethyl-phenylhydrazine, glycyrrhetinic acid, p-hydrazinobenzoic acid, isosafrole, kaempferol, dl-menthol, nicotine, norharman, phenethyl isothiocyanate, pilocarpine, piperidine, protocatechuic acid, rotenone, rutin sulfate, sodium benzoate, tannic acid, 1-trans-δ^9-tetrahydrocannabinol, turmeric oleoresin, vinblastine

The 38 rodent carcinogens listed at the top of the table occur in:

absinthe, allspice, anise, apple, apricot, banana, basil, beet, broccoli, Brussels sprouts, cabbage, cantaloupe, caraway, cardamom, carrot, cauliflower, celery, cherries, chili pepper, chocolate, cinnamon, citronella, cloves, coffee, collard greens, comfrey herb tea, corn, coriander, currants, dill, eggplant, endive, fennel, garlic, grapefruit, grapes, guava, honey, honeydew melon, horseradish, kale, lemon, lentils, lettuce, licorice, lime, mace, mango, marjoram, mint, mushrooms, mustard, nutmeg, onion, orange, oregano, paprika, parsley, parsnip, peach, pear, peas, black pepper, pineapple, plum, potato, radish, raspberries, rhubarb, rosemary, rutabaga, sage, savory, sesame seeds, soybean, star anise, tarragon, tea, thyme, tomato, turmeric, and turnip.

Source: **Carcinogenic Potency Database** (http://potency.berkeley.edu; Gold & al. 1999; Gold & Zeiger 1997).
Note: Fungal toxins are not included.

Table 3: Carcinogenicity in rodents of natural chemicals in roasted coffee

Carcinogens: **N = 21**	acetaldehyde, benzaldehyde, benzene, benzofuran, benzo(*a*)pyrene, caffeic acid, catechol, 1,2,5,6-dibenzanthracene, ethanol, ethylbenzene, formaldehyde, furan, furfural, hydrogen peroxide, hydroquinone, isoprene, limonene, 4-methylcatechol, styrene, toluene, xylene
Noncarcinogens: **N = 8**	acrolein, biphenyl, choline, eugenol, nicotinamide, nicotinic acid, phenol, piperidine
Uncertain:	caffeine
Yet to test:	about 1000 chemicals

Source: ***Carcinogenic Potency Database*** (http://potency.berkeley.edu; Gold & al. 1999; Gold & Zeiger 1997).

Misconception 5—The toxicology of synthetic chemicals is different from that of natural chemicals

It is often assumed that, because natural chemicals are part of human evolutionary history whereas synthetic chemicals are recent, the mechanisms that have evolved in animals to cope with the toxicity of natural chemicals will fail to protect against synthetic chemicals (Ames & al. 1987, Letters). This assumption is flawed for several reasons (Ames & al. 1996; Ames & al. 1990b; Gold & al. 1997b).

Natural defenses are general rather than specific for each chemical

Humans have many natural defenses that buffer against normal exposures to toxins (Ames & al. 1990b); these usually are general rather than tailored to each specific chemical. Thus, the defenses work against both natural and synthetic chemicals. Examples of general defenses include the continuous shedding of cells exposed to toxins—the surface layers of the mouth, esophagus, stomach, intestine, colon, skin, and lungs are discarded every few days; DNA repair enzymes, which repair DNA that has been damaged from many different sources; and detoxification enzymes of the liver and other organs, which generally target classes of toxins rather than individual toxins. That defenses are usually general rather than specific for each chemical makes good evolutionary sense. The reason that predators of plants evolved general defenses presumably was to be prepared to counter a diverse and ever-changing array of plant toxins in an evolving world: a herbivore that had defenses against only a set of specific toxins would be at a great disadvantage in obtaining new food when favored foods became scarce or evolved new toxins.

Natural agents can be carcinogenic to humans

Various natural agents that have been present throughout vertebrate evolutionary history nevertheless cause cancer in vertebrates (Ames & al. 1990b; Gold & al. 1999; Gold & al. 1997a; Vainio & al. 1995). Mold toxins, such as aflatoxin, have been shown to cause cancer in rodents and other species, including humans (Gold & al. 1999). Despite their presence throughout evolution, many of the common elements are carcinogenic to humans at high doses (e.g., salts of cadmium, beryllium, nickel, chromium, and arsenic). Furthermore, *epidemiological* studies from various parts of the world show that certain natural chemicals in food may be carcinogenic risks to humans: for example, the chewing of betel nuts with tobacco is associated with oral cancer, and Chinese-style salted fish is associated with nasopharyngeal cancer (Gold & al. 2001a, http://monographs.iarc.fr/monoeval/crthgr01.html).

Humans have not had time to evolve a "toxic harmony" with all of the plants in their diet. The human diet has changed markedly in the last few thousand years. Indeed, very few of the plants that humans eat today (e.g. coffee, cocoa, tea, potatoes, tomatoes, corn, avocados, mangoes, olives, and kiwi fruit) would have been present in a hunter-gatherer's diet. Natural selection works far too slowly for humans to have evolved specific resistance to the food toxins in these relatively newly introduced plants.

Since no plot of land is free from attack by insects, plants need chemical defenses—either natural or synthetic—in order to survive. Thus, there is a trade-off between naturally occurring and synthetic pesticides. One consequence of disproportionate concern about residues from synthetic pesticides is that some plant breeders develop plants that are more insect-resistant because they are higher in natural toxins.

A case study illustrates the potential hazards of this approach to pest control. When a major grower introduced a new variety of highly insect-resistant celery into commerce, people who handled the celery developed rashes when they were subsequently exposed to sunlight. Some detective work found that the pest-resistant celery contained 6200 parts per billion (ppb) of carcinogenic (and mutagenic) psoralens instead of the 800 ppb present in common celery (Berkley & al. 1986; Gold & al. 1999; Gold & al. 1997b).

Misconception 6—Cancer risks to humans can be assessed by standard high-dose animal cancer tests

Approximately half of all chemicals that have been tested in standard animal cancer tests, whether natural or synthetic, are rodent carcinogens (table 4; Gold & al. 1989a; Gold & al. 1999; Gold & al. 1997a). Why do so many test positive? A reasonable explanation is that the design of these experiments produces effects that would not occur at lower doses. In standard cancer tests, rodents are given chronic, near-toxic doses, the maximum tolerated dose (MTD). The rationale for this experimental design was based on a consensus in the 1970s that chemicals with carcinogenic potential would be rare and, therefore, experiments had to be designed to maximize the chance of finding an effect. Since the costs of conducting these tests are high—currently $2 million to $4 million per chemical (US National Toxicology Program 1998)—a limited number of animals would be put on test (50 in each of three groups: the controls, a group receiving a high dose, and a group receiving half the high dose). Because of the small number of animals on test, the studies lack statistical power and, therefore, the doses were set as high as the animals would tolerate while living long enough to get cancer, since cancer is a disease of old age. Evidence is accumulating that cell division

Table 4: Proportion of chemicals evaluated as carcinogenic

Chemicals tested in both rats and mice [a]	
Chemicals in Carcinogenic Potency Database (CPDB)	350/590 (59%)
Naturally occurring chemicals in the CPDB	79/139 (57%)
Synthetic chemicals in the CPDB	271/451 (60%)
Chemicals tested in rats and/or mice [a]	
Chemicals in the CPDB	702/1348 (52%)
Natural pesticides in the CPDB	37/72 (51%)
Mold toxins in the CPDB	14/23 (61%)
Chemicals in roasted coffee in the CPDB	21/30 (70%)
Commercial pesticides	79/194 (41%)
Innes negative chemicals retested [a]	17/34 (50%)
Physician's Desk Reference (PDR): drugs with reported cancer tests [b]	117/241 (49%)
FDA database of drug submissions [c]	125/282 (44%)

Sources: (a) *Carcinogenic Potency Database* (http://potency.berkeley.edu; Gold & al. 1999; Gold & Zeiger 1997); (b) Davies & Monro 1995; (c) Contrera & al. 1997.

Note: 140 drugs are in the databases of both the Food and Drug Administration (FDA) and the *Physician's Desk Reference* (**PDR**).

caused by the high dose itself, rather than the chemical per se, is increasing the carcinogenic effects and, therefore, the positivity rate. High doses can cause chronic wounding of tissues, cell death, and consequent chronic cell division of neighboring cells. This is a risk factor for cancer (Ames & al. 1996) because, each time a cell divides, the probability increases that a mutation will occur, thereby increasing the risk for cancer.

At the low levels to which humans are usually exposed, such increased cell division does not occur. The process of mutagenesis and carcinogenesis is complicated because many factors are involved: e.g. DNA lesions, DNA repair, cell division, clonal instability, apoptosis (cell suicide in response to DNA damage), and p53 (a cell cycle control gene that is mutated in half of human tumors) (Christensen & al. 1999; Hill & al. 1999). The normal endogenous level of *oxidative DNA lesions* in cells is appreciable (Helbock & al. 1998). In addition, tissues injured by high doses of chemicals have an inflammatory immune response involving activation of white cells in response to cell death (Adachi & al. 1995; Czaja & al. 1994; Gunawardhana & al. 1993; Laskin & Pendino 1995; Laskin & al. 1988; Roberts & Kimber 1999; Wei & al. 1993a; Wei & al. 1993b). Activated white cells release mutagenic oxidants (including peroxynitrite, hypochlorite, and H_2O_2). Therefore, the very low levels of chemicals to which humans are exposed through water pollution or synthetic pesticide residues may pose no, or only minimal, cancer risks because these effects do not occur at low doses.

Analyses of the limited data on dose-response in bioassays are consistent with the idea that cell division from cell-killing and cell replacement is important. Among rodent bioassays with two doses and a control group, about half the sites evaluated as target sites are statistically significant at the MTD but not at half the MTD ($p < 0.05$). Ad libitum feeding in the standard bioassay can also contribute to the high positivity rate (Hart & al. 1995a). In mice fed a restricted number of calories, cell division rates are markedly lower in several tissues than in mice fed ad libitum (Lok & al. 1990). Linearity of response to increasing dosage seems less likely than has been assumed because of the *inducibility* of the numerous defense enzymes that deal with exogenous chemicals as groups (e.g. oxidants, electrophiles) and thus protect us against the natural world of mutagens as well as the small amounts of synthetic chemicals to which we are exposed (Ames & al. 1990b; Calabrese & Baldwin 2001; Luckey 1999; Munday & Munday 1999; Trosko 1998).

Risk assessment requires additional biological data

More than a decade ago, we argued that risk assessment for humans requires data on the mechanism of carcinogenesis for each chemical (Ames & Gold 1990; Ames & al. 1987). Historically, standard practice in regulatory risk assessment for chemicals that induce tumors in high-dose rodent bioassays has been to extrapolate risk to low dose in humans by multiplying rodent potency by human exposure, i.e. by assuming linearity in the dose response. Without data on the mechanism of carcinogenesis, however, the true human risk of cancer at low dose is highly uncertain and could be zero (Ames & Gold 1990; Clayson & Iverson 1996; Gold & al. 1992; Goodman 1994). Adequate risk assessment from animal cancer tests requires more information for a chemical, about pharmacokinetics, mechanism of action, apoptosis, cell division, induction of defense and repair systems, and differences among species. Several mechanisms have now been identified that indicate that carcinogenic effects at the high doses of rodent tests would not be relevant to the low doses of most human exposures (e.g. saccharin, BHA, chloroform, *d*-limonene). Under the new *Guidelines for Cancer Risk Assessment* from the US Environmental Protection Agency (EPA), these mechanisms are to be considered in evaluating the dose-response, method of risk assessment, and relevance to humans; the default linear extrapolation has been replaced by this more scientific approach (US Environmental Protection Agency 1999).

Examples of such biologically based mechanisms include cell proliferation following cytotoxic effects at high doses of saccharin, only in the male rat urothelium; the cytotoxicity results from formation of a precipitate in rat urine, which is a species-specific response. For several chemicals, studies show an association between cell division in the rodent liver and cancer (e.g. chloroform, oxazepam, 2,4-diaminotoluene) (Ames & Gold 1990; Ames & al. 1993a; Butterworth & Bogdanffy 1999; Cohen 1998; Cunningham & al. 1994a; Cunningham & al. 1991; Cunningham & al. 1994b; Heddle 1998). Some chemicals (e.g. d-limonene, induce kidney tumors in male rats by a mechanism that is not relevant to humans: accumulation of a male rat-specific protein (α_{2u}-globulin) resulting in toxicity to the kidney, sustained cell proliferation, and kidney tumors. Humans do not synthesize α_{2u}-globulin or any protein that can function like it (Swenberg & Lehman-McKeeman 1999) and, therefore, the carcinogenic effect in male rats is not predictive of a cancer hazard to humans. Some chemicals induce thyroid follicular-cell tumors at high doses by a metabolic inactivation of the thyroid hormones T_3 and T_4, which results in increased levels of thyroid-stimulating hormone levels, sustained proliferation of cells in the thyroid, and tumor formation (McClain 1990). Humans are less sensitive to this secondary, threshold mechanism than rats (McClain 1994; US Environmental Protection Agency 1998a).

The US EPA's evaluation of chloroform provides an example of the new emphasis on incorporating more biological information into evaluations of cancer test results and risk assessment. The EPA concluded that chloroform-induced tumors were secondary to toxic effects that occur at high dose. Therefore, the EPA relied on a nonlinear dose-response approach with a margin of exposure to estimate cancer risk for humans. They concluded that

> chloroform is likely to be carcinogenic to humans by all routes of exposure under high-exposure conditions that lead to cytotoxicity and regenerative hyperplasia in susceptible tissues. Chloroform is not likely to be carcinogenic to humans by any route of exposure under exposure conditions that do not cause cytotoxicity and cell regeneration. (US Environmental Protection Agency 2002)

Is selection bias causing the high positivity rate?

Since the results of high-dose rodent tests are routinely used to identify a chemical as a possible cancer hazard to humans, it is important that we try to understand how representative the 50% positivity rate might be of all untested chemicals. If half of all chemicals (both natural and synthetic) to which humans are exposed would be positive if tested, then the utility of a rodent bioassay to identify a chemical as a "potential human carcinogen" is questionable. To determine the true proportion of rodent carcinogens among chemicals would require a comparison of a random group of synthetic chemicals to a random group of natural chemicals. Such an analysis has not been done.

A counter argument to the idea that the 50% positivity rate is due to the effects of administering high doses is that so many chemicals are positive because they were selected for testing on the grounds that they were expected to be carcinogenic. We have discussed that this is a likely bias since cancer testing is both expensive and time consuming, making it prudent to test suspicious compounds (Gold & al. 1998); however, chemicals are selected for cancer-testing for many reasons other than suspicion, including the extent of human exposure, level of production and occupational exposure, and scientific questions about carcinogenesis. Moreover, if the main basis for selection was that chemicals were suspected carcinogens, then one should select mutagens (80% are carcinogens compared to 49% of nonmutagens); yet, 55% of the chemicals tested are nonmutagens (Gold & al. 1998). The idea that chemicals are selected for testing because they are likely to be carcinogenic, rests on an assumption that researchers have adequate knowledge about how to predict carcinogenicity and that there is consensus about the criteria; that is, the idea that bias in the positivity rate is due to selection requires that there is shared, adequate knowledge of what is likely to be carcinogenic.

However, while some chemical classes are more often carcinogenic in rodent bioassays than others—e.g. nitroso compounds, aromatic amines, nitroaromatics, and chlorinated compounds—several results suggest that predictive knowledge is highly imperfect, even now after decades of testing results on which to base predictions have become available. For example, a prospective prediction exercise was conducted by several experts in 1990 in advance of the 2-year bioassays by the United States National Toxicology Program (NTP). There was wide disagreement among the experts as to which chemicals would be carcinogenic when tested; accuracy varied, thus indicating that predictive knowledge is uncertain (Omenn & al. 1995). One predictive analysis for a randomly selected group of chemicals has been conducted using a computerized method based on chemical structure; among 140 randomly selected chemicals, 65 (46%) were predicted to be carcinogenic if tested in standard bioassays (Rosenkranz & Klopman 1990). Another argument against the hypothesis of selection bias is the high positivity rate for drugs (table 4), because drug development tends to select chemicals that are not mutagens or expected carcinogens.

A study by Innes & al. (1969) has frequently been cited (Ames & al. 1987, Letters) as evidence that the positivity rate is low, because only 9% of 119 chemicals tested (primarily pesticides) were positive. However, the Innes tests were only in mice, had only 18 animals per group, and were terminated at 18 months. This protocol lacked the power of modern experiments, in which both rats and mice are tested, with 50 animals per group for 24 months. When 34 chemicals for which Innes obtained negative results were retested in other strains of mice or in rats, using more adequate protocols including higher doses and longer experiment length, 17 of the 34 formerly negative chemicals tested positive (table 4) (Cohen 1995; Cohen & Lawson 1995; Gold & al. 1999; Gold & al. 1997a).

Thus, it seems likely that a high proportion of all chemicals, whether synthetic or natural, might be "carcinogens" if run through the standard rodent bioassay at the MTD. For nonmutagens, carcinogenicity would be primarily due to the effects of high doses; for mutagens, it would result from a synergistic effect between cell division at high doses and DNA damage (Ames & Gold 1990; Ames & al. 1993a; Butterworth & al. 1995). Without additional data on the mechanism of carcinogenesis for each chemical, the interpretation of a positive result in a rodent bioassay is highly uncertain. The carcinogenic effects may be limited to the high dose tested.

Problems in extrapolating carcinogenicity between species

The use of bioassay results in risk assessment requires a qualitative species extrapolation from rats or mice to humans. The accuracy of this extrapolation is generally unverifiable, since data on humans are limited. Ultimately one wants to know whether the large number (many hundreds) of chemicals that have been shown to be carcinogenic in experimental animals would also be carcinogenic in humans. This question cannot be answered by reversing the question—that is, by asking whether the small number of chemicals that are carcinogenic to humans are also carcinogenic in rodent bioassays—because, even if most human carcinogens were carcinogenic to experimental animals, the converse does not necessarily follow, as can be demonstrated by a simple probabilistic argument (Freedman & Zeisel 1988).

Evidence about interspecies extrapolation can, however, be obtained by investigating whether chemicals that are carcinogenic in rats are also carcinogenic in mice, and visa versa. If mice and rats are similar with respect to carcinogenesis, this provides some evidence in favor of interspecies extrapolations; conversely, if mice and rats are different, this casts doubt on the validity of extrapolations from mice to humans.

One measure of interspecies agreement is concordance, the percentage of chemicals that are classified the same way as to carcinogenicity in mice and rats (i.e. results are concordant if a chemical is a carcinogen in either both species or in neither, and results are discordant if a chemical is a carcinogen in one species but not in the other). Observed concordance in bioassays is about 75% (Gold & al. 1997a; Gold & al. 1998), which may seem low since the experimental conditions are identical and the species are similar. The observed concordance is just an estimate based on limited data. We have shown by simulations for 300 *NCI/NTP* bioassays of chemicals tested in both rats and mice (which have an observed concordance of 75%), that an observed concordance of 75% can arise if the true concordance is anything between 20% and 100% (Freedman & al. 1996; Lin & al. 1995) and, indeed, observed concordance can seriously overestimate true concordance. Thus, it seems unlikely that true concordance between rats and mice can be estimated with any reasonable degree of confidence from bioassay data.

Problems in using results of animal cancer tests for regulatory risk assessment

We have discussed the problems in deriving valid human risk assessments from the limited data from animal cancer tests (Bernstein & al. 1985; Gold & al. 1998). Standard practice in regulatory risk assessment for a given rodent carcinogen has been to extrapolate from the high doses of rodent bioassays to the low doses of most human exposures by multiplying *carcinogenic potency* in rodents by human exposure. Strikingly, however, due to the relatively narrow range of doses in 2-year rodent bioassays and the limited range of statistically significant tumor incidence rates, the various measures of potency obtained from 2-year bioassays, such as the EPA's q_1^* value, the TD_{50}, and the lower confidence limit on the TD_{10} (LTD_{10}) are constrained to a relatively narrow range of values about the MTD, in the absence of 100% tumor incidence at the target site, which rarely occurs (Bernstein & al. 1985; Freedman & al. 1993; Gaylor & Gold 1995; Gaylor & Gold 1998; Gold & al. 1997a). For example, the dose usually estimated by regulatory agencies to give one cancer in a million can be approximated simply by using the MTD as a surrogate for carcinogenic potency. Gaylor and Gold (1995) have shown that the "virtually safe dose" (VSD) can be approximated by the MTD/740,000 for rodent carcinogens tested in the bioassay program of the NCI/NTP. The MTD/740,000 was within a factor of 10 of the VSD for 96% of carcinogens. This is similar to the finding that in near-replicate experiments of the same chemical, potency estimates vary by a factor of 4 around a median value (Gaylor & al. 1993; Gold & al. 1989b; Gold & al. 1987b).

Using the benchmark dose approach proposed in the EPA carcinogen guidelines, risk estimation is similarly constrained by bioassay design. A simple, quick, and relatively precise determination of the LTD_{10} can be obtained by the maximum tolerated dose (MTD) divided by 7 (Gaylor &

Gold 1998). Both linear extrapolation and the use of safety or uncertainty factors proportionately reduce a tumor dose in a similar manner. The difference in the regulatory "safe dose," if any, for the two approaches depends on the magnitude of uncertainty factors selected. Using the benchmark dose approach of the proposed carcinogen risk assessment guidelines, the dose estimated from the LTD_{10} divided, for example, by a 1000-fold uncertainty factor is similar to the dose of an estimated risk of less than 10^{-4} using a linear model. This dose is 100 times higher than the VSD corresponding to an estimated risk of less than 10^{-6}. Thus, whether the procedure involves a benchmark dose or a linearized model, cancer risk estimation is constrained by the bioassay design.

Misconception 7—Synthetic chemicals pose greater carcinogenic hazards than natural chemicals

An analysis of synthetic chemicals against the vast array of natural chemicals shows that synthetic rodent carcinogens are a tiny fraction of the total. In several papers (Ames & al. 1995; Ames & al. 1987; Ames & al. 1990a; Gold & al. 1999; Gold & al. 1992), we have emphasized the importance of setting research and regulatory priorities by gaining a broad perspective about the vast number of chemicals to which humans are exposed. A comparison of potential hazards using a simple index can be helpful in efforts to communicate what might be important factors in cancer prevention and when selecting chemicals for *chronic bioassay*, mechanistic, or *epidemiologic* studies (Ames & al. 1987; Ames & al. 1990b; Gold & al. 1992; Gold & Zeiger 1997). There is a need to identify what might be the important cancer hazards among the ubiquitous exposures to rodent carcinogens in everyday life.

Human Exposure/Rodent Potency index (HERP)—ranking possible human cancer hazards from rodent carcinogens

One reasonable strategy for setting priorities is to use a rough index to compare and rank possible carcinogenic hazards from a wide variety of chemical exposures at levels that humans typically receive, and then to focus on those that rank highest (Gold & al. 1999; Gold & al. 1997a; Gold & al. 1992). Ranking is thus a critical first step. Although one cannot say whether the ranked chemical exposures are likely to be of major or minor importance in human cancer, it is not prudent to focus attention on the possible hazards at the bottom of a ranking if, by using the same methodology to identify hazard, there are numerous common human exposures with much greater possible hazards. Research on the mechanism of carcinogenesis for a given chemical is needed to interpret the possible human risk. The ranking of possible hazards is in table 5, pp. 71–85. A description of the fields is on p. 71. Our analyses are based on the Human Exposure/ Rodent Potency index (**HERP**), which indicates what percentage of the rodent carcinogenic potency (**TD_{50}** in mg/kg/ day) a person receives from a given average daily dose when exposed over a lifetime (mg/kg/day) (Gold & Zeiger 1997). The method for calculating the HERP index, including an example, is described in the **Appendix** (p. 97). TD_{50} values in our CPDB span a 10 million-fold range across chemicals (Gold & al. 1997c). Human exposures to rodent carcinogens range enormously as well, from historically high workplace exposures in some occupations or pharmaceutical dosages to very low exposures from residues of synthetic chemicals in food or water. Consideration of both these values for a chemical is necessary for ranking possible hazard.

Overall, our HERP ranking has shown that synthetic pesticide residues rank low in possible carcinogenic hazard compared to many common exposures. HERP values for some historically high exposures in the workplace and some pharmaceuticals rank high, and there is an enormous background of naturally occurring rodent carcinogens in average consumption of common foods. This background of natural chemical results casts doubt on the relative importance of low-dose exposures to residues of synthetic chemicals such as pesticides (Ames & al. 1987; Gold & al. 1994a; Gold & al.

1992). A committee of the National Research Council recently reached similar conclusions when they compared natural and synthetic chemicals in the diet and called for further research on natural chemicals (National Research Council 1996). The rank order of possible hazards by HERP is similar to the order that would be based on a linear model.

The ranking of possible hazards (HERP values in %) in table 5 (pp. 71–85) is for average exposures in the United States to all rodent carcinogens in the CPDB for which concentration data and average United States exposure or consumption data were both available, and for which human exposure could be chronic for a lifetime. For pharmaceuticals, the doses are recommended doses, and for exposure in the workplace they are past averages for an industry or a high-exposure occupation. The 94 exposures in the ranking (table 5) are ordered by possible carcinogenic hazard (HERP) and natural chemicals in the diet are reported in boldface. Several HERP values make convenient reference points for interpreting table 5. The median HERP value is 0.002% and the background HERP for the average chloroform level in a liter of United States tap water is 0.0008%. Chloroform is formed as a by-product of water chlorination and the HERP value reflects exposure to chloroform from both drinking water and breathing indoor air, for example, when showering (chloroform is volatile.). A HERP of 0.00001% is approximately equal to a regulatory risk level of 1-in-a-million based on a linear model, i.e. the Virtually Safe Dose (VSD) (Gold & al. 1992). The rank order in table 5 would be the same for a Margin of Exposure (MOE) from the TD_{50} because the MOE is inversely related to HERP.

Table 5 indicates that, if the same methodology were used for both naturally occurring and synthetic chemicals, most ordinary foods would not pass the default regulatory criteria that have been used for synthetic chemicals. For many natural chemicals, the HERP values are in the top half of the table, even though natural chemicals are markedly under-represented because so few have been tested in rodent bioassays. The ranking of HERP values maximizes possible hazards from synthetic chemicals because it includes historically high exposure values that are now much lower, for example, exposure to DDT and saccharin as well as to occupational chemicals.

For readers who are interested in the results for particular categories of exposure or particular chemicals, we discuss below several categories of exposure and selected chemicals. We indicate for some chemicals the mechanistic data suggesting that the rodent results may not be relevant to humans or that possible hazards would be lower if non-linearity or a threshold in the dose-response were taken into account in risk assessment.

Occupational exposures

Occupational exposures to some chemicals have been high and many of the single chemical agents or industrial processes evaluated as human carcinogens have been identified by historically high exposures in the workplace (International Agency for Research on Cancer 1971–2002; Tomatis & Bartsch 1990). HERP values rank at or near the top of table 5 for highly exposed occupational groups, mostly from the past: ethylene dibromide, 1,3-butadiene, tetrachloroethylene, formaldehyde, acrylonitrile, trichloroethylene, and methylene chloride. The assessment of exposure in occupational settings is often difficult because workers are often exposed occupationally to more than one chemical at a time or over the course of a worklife. Epidemiological studies are often small and lack information on potentially *confounding factors* such as smoking and alcohol consumption. The International Agency for Research on Cancer (IARC) has evaluated the evidence in humans as limited for butadiene, trichloroethylene, tetrachloroethylene, and formaldehyde; for ethylene dibromide, acrylonitrile, and methylene chloride the evidence is inadequate (International Agency for Research on Cancer 1971–2002). Unlike the IARC, the National Toxicology Program (US National Toxicology Program 2000b) considered 1,3-butadiene to be a human carcinogen; the two agencies differed with respect to their evaluation of the strength of evidence for leukemia in workers exposed to butadiene and in whether an increased risk in the styrene-butadiene industry may have been due to exposures other than butadiene (International Agency for Research on Cancer 1999a; US National Toxicology Program 2000b). The rodent carcinogens listed in the HERP table as occupational exposures also occur naturally, with the exception of ethylene dibromide: for example, butadiene occurs in forest fires, environmental tobacco smoke, and heated cooking oils (Shields & al. 1995); acrylonitrile occurs in cigarette smoke; formaldehyde is ubiquitous in food, is generated metabolically in animals, and is present in human blood.

The possible hazard estimated for past actual exposure levels of workers most heavily exposed to ethylene dibromide (EDB) is the highest in table 5 (HERP = 140%). We testified in 1981 that our calculations showed that the workers were allowed to breathe in a dose higher than the dose that gave half of the test rats cancer, although the level of human exposure may have been somewhat overestimated (California Department of Health Services 1985). An epidemiologic study of these workers, who inhaled EDB for over a decade, did not show any increase in cancer; however, because of the relatively small numbers of people tested the study lacked the statistical power to detect a small effect (California Department of Health Services 1985; Ott & al. 1980; Ramsey & al. 1978). Ethylene dibromide is no longer produced in the United States and nearly all of its uses have been discontinued (the primary use was as an antiknock agent in leaded gasoline).

For trichloroethylene (TCE), the HERP is 2.2% for workers (vapor degreasers) who cleaned equipment with

TCE prior to 1977. We recently conducted an analysis (Bogen & Gold 1997) based on the assumption that carcinogenic effects are due to toxic effects from peak doses to the liver, the target organ for trichloroethylene carcinogenicity in mice. Our estimates indicate that for occupational respiratory exposures, the Permissible Exposure Limit (PEL) for trichloroethylene would produce concentrations of TCE metabolites that are higher than the no observed effect level (NOEL) for liver toxicity in mice. On this basis, the PEL is not expected to be protective. In contrast, the EPA's maximum concentration limit (MCL) in drinking water of 5 µg/liter based on a linearized multistage model is more stringent than our safe-dose estimate based on a 1000-fold safety factor, which is 210 µg/liter (Bogen & Gold 1997).

In other analyses, we used PELs of the United States Occupational Safety and Health Administration (OSHA) as surrogates for actual exposures and compared the permitted daily dose-rate for workers with the TD_{50} in rodents (PERP index, Permissible Exposure/Rodent Potency) (Gold & al. 1987a; Gold & al. 1994a) For current permitted levels, PERP values for 14 chemicals are greater than 10%. Because workers can be exposed chronically to high doses of chemicals, it is important to have protective exposure limits (Gold & al. 1994a). In recent years, the permitted exposures for 1,3-butadiene and methylene chloride have been lowered substantially in the United States, and the current PERP values are below 1%.

Pharmaceuticals and herbal supplements

In table 4, we reported that half the drugs in the *Physician's Desk Reference* (PDR) that have reported cancer test data are carcinogens in rodent bioassays (Davies & Monro 1995), as are 44% of drug submissions to United States Food and Drug Administration (FDA) (Contrera & al. 1997). Most drugs, however, are used only for short periods and, therefore, we have not calculated HERP values for them. Pharmaceuticals

Misconceptions about the Causes of Cancer

are evaluated by the FDA using mechanistic data as well as tumor incidence, and taking benefits into account.

The HERP ranking includes pharmaceuticals that can be used chronically; some are high in the HERP ranking, primarily because the dose ingested is high. Phenobarbital (HERP = 12%) is a sedative and anticonvulsant that has been investigated in humans who took it for decades; there is no convincing evidence that it caused cancer (American Medical Association Division of Drugs 1983; Freidman & Habel 1999; McLean & al. 1986). Mechanistic data suggest that the dose-response curve for tumors induced in rodents is nonlinear and perhaps exhibits a threshold.

Four cholesterol-lowering drugs have evidence of carcinogenicity in rodent tests; they are not mutagenic or genotoxic and long-term epidemiological studies and clinical trials have not provided evidence of an association with fatal or non-fatal cancers in humans (Bjerre & LeLorier 2001; Childs & Girardot 1992; Havel & Kane 1982; International Agency for Research on Cancer 1996; Pfeffer & al. 2002; Reddy & Lalwani 1983; World Health Organization 1984). Two of these drugs, clofibrate (HERP = 17%), which was used as a cholesterol-lowering agent primarily before the 1970s, and gemfibrozil (HERP = 6.9%), which is currently used, increase liver tumors in rodents by the mechanism of peroxisome proliferation. This suggests that they would not be expected to be carcinogenic in humans (Cattley & al. 1996; Havel & Kane 1982; Reddy & Lalwani 1983; World Health Organization 1984). The two other cholesterol-lowering drugs in table 5 are statins: fluvastatin (HERP = 0.2%) and the widely-used drug, lovastatin (HERP = 0.06%). Large clinical trials of statins have shown no carcinogenic effects in humans, although there were limitations in the studies: the follow-up period of 5 years is short for observing carcinogenic effects and the trials were not designed to measure cancer risk (Bjerre & LeLorier 2001; Guallar & Goodman 2001; Pfeffer & al. 2002). A meta-analysis of 5 clinical trials examined only the combination of all cancers rather than specific types of cancer (Guallar & Goodman 2001).

Herbal supplements have recently developed into a large market in the United States; they have not been a focus of carcinogenicity testing. The FDA regulatory requirements for safety and efficacy that are applied to pharmaceuticals do not apply to herbal supplements under the 1994 Dietary Supplement and Health Education Act (DSHEA) and few have been tested for carcinogenicity. The relevant regulatory requirements in Canada are under review and current regulations treat non-prescription ingredients of botanical origin separately from pharmaceuticals (Health Canada 1995; Volpe 1998). Those that are rodent carcinogens tend to rank high in HERP because, like some pharmaceutical drugs, the recommended dose is high relative to the rodent carcinogenic dose. Moreover, under DSHEA the safety criteria that have been used for decades by FDA for food additives that are "Generally Recognized As Safe" (GRAS) are not applicable to dietary supplements (Burdock 2000), even though supplements are used at higher doses. The *NTP* is currently testing several medicinal herbs or chemicals that are present in herbs.

Comfrey
Comfrey is a medicinal herb whose roots and leaves have been shown to be carcinogenic in rats. For the formerly recommended dose of 9 daily comfrey-pepsin tablets, HERP = 6.2%. Symphytine, a pyrrolizidine-alkaloid that is a natural plant pesticide, is a rodent carcinogen present in comfrey-pepsin tablets and comfrey tea. The HERP value for symphytine is 1.3% in the pills and 0.03% in comfrey herb tea. Comfrey pills are no longer widely sold but are available on the World Wide Web. Comfrey roots and leaves can be bought at health-food stores and on the Web and can thus be used for tea, although comfrey is recommended for topical use only in the *PDR for Herbal Medicines* (Gruenwald &

al. 1998). Poisoning epidemics by pyrrolizidine alkaloids have occurred in the developing world. In the United States, poisonings, including deaths, have been associated with use of herbal teas containing comfrey (Huxtable 1995). Recently, the US FDA issued a warning about comfrey and asked manufacturers to withdraw their comfrey products after several people became ill from taking comfrey as a supplement or as tea. Comfrey is banned from distribution in Canada (Stickel & Seitz 2000). Several other medicinal plants containing pyrrolizidine are rodent carcinogens, including coltsfoot, *Senecio longilobus* and *S. nemorensis*, *Petasites japonicus*, and *Farfugium japonicum*. Over 200 pyrrolizidine alkaloids are present in more than 300 plant species. Up to 3% of flowering plant species contain pyrrolizidine alkaloids (Prakash & al. 1999). Several pyrrolizidine alkaloids have been tested chronically in rodent bioassays and are carcinogenic (Gold & al. 1997c).

Dehydroepiandrosterone (DHEA)

Dehydroepiandrosterone (DHEA) and DHEA sulfate are the major secretion products of adrenal glands in humans and are precursors of androgenic and estrogenic hormones (Oelkers 1999; van Vollenhoven 2000). DHEA is manufactured as a dietary supplement, and sold widely for a variety of purposes including the delay of aging. DHEA is a controlled drug in Canada (Health Canada 2000). In rats, DHEA induces liver tumors (Hayashi & al. 1994; Rao & al. 1992) and the HERP value for the recommended human dose of one daily capsule containing 25 mg DHEA is 0.5%. Peroxisome proliferation is the mechanism of liver carcinogenesis in rats for DHEA, suggesting that the carcinogenicity may not be relevant to humans (Hayashi & al. 1994). DHEA inhibited the development of tumors of the rat testis (Rao 1992) and the rat and mouse mammary gland (McCormick & al. 1996; Schwartz & al. 1981). A recent review of clinical, experimental, and epidemiological studies concluded that late promotion of breast cancer in postmenopausal women may be stimulated by prolonged intake of DHEA (Stoll 1999); however the evidence for a positive association in postmenopausal women between serum DHEA levels and breast cancer risk is conflicting (Bernstein & al. 1990; Stoll 1999).

Aristolochic acid
Herbal medicinal products containing aristolochic acid have been found to induce cancer in the urinary tracts of humans and the FDA has issued warnings about supplements and traditional medicines that contain aristolochic acid (Schwetz 2001, http://www.cfsan.fda.gov/%20~dms/ds-bot.html). *Aristolochia* species, which are the source of aristolochic acid, are listed in the Chinese pharmacopoeia (Reid 1993). In a diet clinic in Belgium, aristolochic acid was unintentionally administered to patients in pills which purportedly contained a chemical from a different plant species. Many of the female patients who took aristolochic acid developed kidney disease (**Chinese-herb nephropathy**), and the cumulative dose of aristolochic acid was related to the progression of the disease. Thirty-nine patients suffered terminal renal failure and, of these, 18 developed urothelial tract carcinoma (Nortier & al. 2000). The average treatment time in the diet clinic was 13.3 months. The mutagenicity and the carcinogenic effects of aristolochic acid in rodent bioassays, was demonstrated two decades ago (Mengs 1982; Mengs 1988; Robisch & al. 1982). In rats, malignant tumors were induced unusually rapidly. No HERP is reported because the human exposures were for a short time only.

Natural pesticides
Natural pesticides, because few have been tested, are markedly underrepresented in our HERP analysis. Importantly, for each plant food listed, there are about 50 additional untested natural pesticides. Although about 10,000 natu-

ral pesticides and their break-down products occur in the human diet (Ames & al. 1990a), only 72 have been tested adequately in rodent bioassays (table 2). Average exposures to many natural pesticides that are carcinogenic in rodents found in common foods rank above or close to the median in the HERP Table, ranging up to a HERP of 0.1%. These include caffeic acid (in coffee, lettuce, tomato, apple, potato, celery, carrot, plum and pear); safrole (in spices and formerly in natural root beer before it was banned), allyl isothiocyanate (mustard), d-limonene (mango, orange juice, black pepper); coumarin in cinnamon; and hydroquinone, catechol, and 4-methylcatechol in coffee. Some natural pesticides in the commonly eaten mushroom (*Agaricus bisporus*) are rodent carcinogens (glutamyl-p-hydrazinobenzoate, p-hydrazinobenzoate), and the HERP based on feeding whole mushrooms to mice is 0.02%. For d-limonene, no human risk is anticipated because tumors are induced only in male rat kidney tubules with involvement of α_{2u}-globulin nephrotoxicity, which does not appear to be relevant for humans (Hard & Whysner 1994; International Agency for Research on Cancer 1993; Rice & al. 1999; US Environmental Protection Agency 1991c).

Synthetic pesticides
Synthetic pesticides currently in use that are rodent carcinogens in the CPDB and that are quantitatively detected by the FDA's Total Diet Study (*TDS*) as residues in food, are all included in Table 5. Several are at the very bottom of the ranking; however, HERP values are about at the median for 3 exposures prior to discontinuance or reduction in use: ethylene thiourea (ETU), toxaphene before its cancellation in the United States in 1982, and DDT before its ban in the United States in 1972. These 3 synthetic pesticides rank below the HERP values for many naturally occurring chemicals that are common in the diet. The HERP values in table 5 are for residue intake by females 65 and older, since

they consume higher amounts of fruits and vegetables than other adult groups, thus maximizing the exposure estimate to pesticide residues. We note that for pesticide residues in the TDS, the consumption estimates for children (mg/kg/day from 1986 to 1991) are within a factor of 3 of the adult consumption (mg/kg/day), greater in adults for some pesticides and greater in children for others (US Food and Drug Administration 1993b).

DDT and other pesticides

DDT and similar early pesticides have been a concern because of their unusual lipophilicity and persistence; however, natural pesticides can also bioaccumulate. There is no convincing epidemiological evidence of a carcinogenic hazard of DDT to humans (Key & Reeves 1994). In a recently completed 24-year study in which DDT was fed to rhesus and cynomolgus monkeys for 11 years, DDT was not evaluated as carcinogenic (Takayama & al. 1999; Thorgeirsson & al. 1994), despite doses that were toxic to both liver and central nervous system. However, the protocol used few animals and dosing was discontinued after 11 years, which may have reduced the sensitivity of the study (Gold & al. 1999).

Current exposure in the United States to DDT and its metabolites is in foods of animal origin and the HERP value is low, 0.00008%. DDT is often viewed as the typically dangerous synthetic pesticide because it concentrates in adipose tissue and persists for years. DDT was the first synthetic pesticide; it eradicated malaria from many parts of the world, including the United States, and was effective against many vectors of disease such as mosquitoes, tsetse flies, lice, ticks and fleas. DDT prevented many millions of deaths from malaria (Jukes 1974). It was also lethal to many crop pests and significantly increased the supply, and lowered the cost, of fresh, nutritious foods, thus making them accessible to more people. DDT was also of low toxicity to humans. There is no convincing epidemiological evidence, nor is there much toxicological plausibility, that the levels of DDT normally found in the environment or in human tissues are likely to be a significant contributor to human cancer (Laden & al. 2001). A recent study of breast cancer on Long Island found no association between breast cancer and blood levels of DDT, DDE, dieldrin or chlordane (Gammon & al. 2002).

DDT is unusual with respect to bioconcentration and, because of its chlorine substituents, it takes longer to degrade in nature than most chemicals; however, these are properties of relatively few synthetic chemicals. In addition, many thousands of chlorinated chemicals are produced in nature (Gribble 1996). Natural pesticides can also bioconcentrate if they are fat-soluble. Potatoes, for example, naturally contain the fat soluble neurotoxins solanine and chaconine (Ames & al. 1990a; Gold & al. 1997b), which can be detected in the bloodstream of all potato eaters. High levels of these potato neurotoxins have been shown to cause birth defects in rodents (Ames & al. 1990b).

The HERP value for ethylene thiourea (ETU), a breakdown product of certain fungicides, is the highest among the synthetic pesticide residues (0.002%), at the median of the ranking. The HERP value would be about 10 times lower if the potency value of the EPA were used instead of our TD_{50}; the EPA combined rodent results from more than one experiment, including one in which ETU was administered in utero, and obtained a weaker potency (US Environmental Protection Agency 1992a). (The CPDB does not include in utero exposures.) Additionally, the EPA has recently discontinued some uses of fungicides for which ETU is a breakdown product and exposure levels are therefore lower.

In 1984, the EPA banned the agricultural use of ethylene dibromide (EDB), the main fumigant in the United States, because of the residue levels found in grain. The HERP value of EDB before the ban (HERP = 0.0004%) ranks low, whereas the HERP of 140% for the high exposures to

EDB that some workers received in the 1970s is at the top of the ranking (Gold & al. 1992). Two other pesticides in table 5, toxaphene (HERP = 0.001% in 1982 and 0.0001% in 1990) and chlorobenzilate (HERP=0.0000001%), have been cancelled (Ames & Gold 1991; US Environmental Protection Agency 1998b).

HERP values for other pesticide residues are all below the median of 0.002%. In descending order of HERP values, these are DDE (before the 1972 ban of DDT), ethylene dibromide, carbaryl, toxaphene (after cancellation), DDE/DDT (after the ban), dicofol, lindane, PCNB, chlorobenzilate, captan, folpet, and chlorothalonil. Some of the lowest HERP values in table 5 are for the synthetic pesticides, captan, chlorothalonil, and folpet, which were also evaluated in 1987 by the National Research Council (NRC) and were considered by NRC to have a human cancer risk above 10^{-6} (National Research Council 1987).

Why were the EPA risk estimates reported by NRC so high when the HERP values are so low? We have investigated this disparity in cancer risk estimates for pesticide residues in the diet by examining the two components of risk assessment: carcinogenic potency estimates from rodent bioassays and human exposure estimates (Gold & al. 2001b; Gold & al. 1997d). We found that potency estimates based on rodent bioassay data are similar whether calculated, as in the NRC report, as the EPA's regulatory q_1^* value or as the TD_{50} in the CPDB. In contrast, estimates of dietary exposure to residues of synthetic pesticides vary enormously, depending on whether they are based on the Theoretical Maximum Residue Contribution (TMRC) calculated by the EPA or the average dietary residues measured by the FDA in the Total Diet Study (TDS). The EPA's TMRC is the theoretical maximum human exposure anticipated under the most severe field application conditions, which is often a large overestimate compared to the measured residues. For several pesticides, the NRC's risk estimate was greater than one in a million whereas the FDA did not detect any residues in the TDS even though the TDS measures residues as low as 1 ppb (Gold & al. 1997d).

In the 1980s, enormous attention was given in the news media to Alar, a chemical used to regulate the growth of apples while on the tree (it is not a pesticide). UDMH, a rodent carcinogen, is the breakdown product of Alar in apples, applesauce, and apple juice (Ames & Gold 1989). The HERP value before use of Alar was discontinued, was 0.001%, just below the median of table 5. Many natural dietary chemicals that are rodent carcinogens have higher HERP values: for example, caffeic acid in lettuce, tomato, apple, and celery; safrole in spices, and catechol in coffee. Apple juice contains 353 natural volatile chemicals (Nijssen & al. 1996), of which only 12 have been tested for carcinogenicity in the CPDB; 9 of these have been found to be carcinogenic.

Cooking and preparation of food

Cooking and preparation of food (e.g. fermentation) also produce chemicals that are rodent carcinogens.

Alcoholic beverages

Alcoholic beverages cause cancer in humans in the liver, esophagus, and oral cavity. Epidemiological studies indicate that all types of alcoholic beverages are associated with increased cancer risk, suggesting that ethyl alcohol itself causes the effect rather than any particular type of beverage. The HERP values in table 5 for alcohol are high in the ranking: HERP = 3.6% for average American consumption of all alcoholic averages combined, 1.8% in beer, and 0.6% in wine.

Cooking food is also plausible as a contributor to cancer as a wide variety of chemicals are formed during cooking. Rodent carcinogens formed during cooking include furfural and similar furans, nitrosamines, polycyclic hydrocarbons, and heterocyclic amines. Furfural, a chemical formed naturally when sugars are heated, is a widespread constituent of food flavor. The HERP value for naturally occurring furfural in average consumption of coffee is 0.006% and, of white bread, is 0.004%.

Acrylamide

Recently, an industrial chemical that is also formed in cigarette smoke, was identified as a common constituent in the human diet. Acrylamide is formed when carbohydrate is cooked at high temperatures; the highest concentrations are in potato chips and French fries (Tareke & al. 2002). Epidemiological studies in workers have not shown an association with cancer (Collins & al. 1989; Marsh & al. 1999). Acrylamide is carcinogenic at several target sites in rat bioassays and the TD_{50} in rats is 8.89 mg/kg/day. No estimates are available for average American consumption; therefore, it is not included in the HERP table (table 5). The estimate for average consumption of dietary acrylamide in Sweden is 40 µg/day (Tareke & al. 2002, http://www.slv.se/engdefault.asp) and the HERP value would be 0.01%. This HERP value is similar to other natural constituents of food such as safrole and furfural. Acrylamide is genotoxic and the HERP value is above the median. This suggests that further work to assess its potential hazard to humans is needed, including further study of the formation and fate of acrylamide in food during cooking and processing, absorption, metabolism, and disposition in humans of acrylamide from food, of the mode of action in the animal cancer tests, and the mechanisms of action and its dose-response characteristics.

Nitrosamines

Nitrosamines are formed in food from nitrite or nitrogen oxides (NO_x) and amines in food. Tobacco smoking and smokeless tobacco are a major source of non-occupational exposure to nitrosamines that are rodent carcinogens: N´-nitrosonornicotine and 4-(methylnitrosamino)-1-(3-pyridyl)-1-(butanone) (Hecht & Hoffmann 1998). Most exposure to nitrosamines in the diet is for chemicals that are not carcinogenic in rodents (Hecht & Hoffmann 1998; Lijinsky 1999). The nitrosamines that are carcinogenic are potent carcinogens (table 5), and it has been estimated that in several countries humans are exposed to about 0.3–1.0 µg per day (Tricker & Preussmann 1991) (National Academy of Sciences, 1981), primarily N-nitrosodimethylamine (DMN), N-nitrosopyrrolidine (NPYR) and N-nitrosopiperidine. The largest exposure was to DMN in beer: concentrations declined more than 30-fold after 1979 (HERP = 0.01%), when it was reported that DMN was formed by the direct-fired drying of malt and the industry modified the process to indirect firing (Glória, Barbour, & Scanlan 1997). By the 1990s, HERP = 0.0002% (Glória & al. 1997). The HERP values for average consumption of bacon are: DMN = 0.0008%, N-Nitrosodiethylamine (DEN) = 0.001%, and NPYR = 0.0007%. DEN induced liver tumors in rhesus and cynomolgus monkeys and tumors of the nasal mucosa in bush babies (Thorgeirsson, & al., 1994). In a study of DMN in rhesus monkeys, no tumors were induced; however, the administered doses produced toxic hepatitis and all animals died early. Thus, the test was not sensitive because the animals may not have lived long enough to develop tumors (Gold & al. 1999; Thorgeirsson & al. 1994).

Heterocyclic amines

A variety of mutagenic and carcinogenic heterocyclic amines (HA) are formed when meat, chicken, or fish is cooked, particularly when charred. HA are potent mutagens with strong evidence of carcinogenicity in terms of positivity rates, multiplicity of species, and target sites; however, concordance in target sites between rats and mice for these HA is generally restricted to the liver (Gold & al. 1994b). Some of the target sites of HA in rats are among the more common cancer sites in humans: colon, prostate, and breast.

Prostate tumors were induced by **PhIP** at only the highest dose tested (400 ppm) and not by other HA (Takahashi & al. 1998). Under usual cooking conditions, exposures to HA are in the low ppb range and the HERP values are low. The values in table 5, which rank below the median, are based on hamburger consumption because hamburger has the best available concentration estimates based on various degrees of doneness. A recent estimate of HA in the total diet was about 2-fold higher than our consumption estimates for hamburger (Bogen & Keating 2001; Keating & Bogen 2001).

For HA in pan-fried hamburger, the HERP value is highest for PhIP, 0.0002%, compared to 0.00003% for **MeIQx** and 0.00001% for **IQ**. Carcinogenicity of the three HA in the HERP table, IQ, MeIQx, and PhIP, has been investigated in studies in cynomolgus monkeys. IQ rapidly induced a high incidence of hepatocellular carcinoma (Adamson & al. 1994) and the HERP value would be 2.5 times higher in monkeys than it would be in rats. MeIQx, which induced tumors at multiple sites in rats and mice (Gold & al. 1997c), did not induce tumors in monkeys (Ogawa & al. 1999). The PhIP study is still in progress. Metabolism studies indicate the importance of N-hydroxylation in the carcinogenic effect of HA in monkeys (Ogawa & al. 1999; Snyderwine & al. 1997).

Food additives

Food additives that are rodent carcinogens can be either naturally occurring (e.g. allyl isothiocyanate, furfural) or synthetic (e.g. butylated hydroxyanisole [BHA] and saccharin). The highest HERP values for average dietary exposures to synthetic rodent carcinogens in table 5 are for exposures in the early 1970s to BHA (0.01%) and saccharin in the 1970s (0.005%). Both are nongenotoxic rodent carcinogens for which data on mechanism of carcinogenesis strongly suggest that there would be no risk to humans at the levels found in food (See **Saccharin** below).

Naturally occurring food additives

For five naturally occurring rodent carcinogens that are also produced commercially and used as food additives, average exposure data were available and they are included in table 5. The HERP value for the natural occurrence of each chemical is greater than for use as a commercial additive because the natural exposures are greater. For furfural (a product of cooking discussed above), the HERP value for the natural occurrence is 0.03% compared to 0.0003% for the additive; for d-limonene, the HERP value is 0.1% for the natural occurrence (e.g. in citrus and other common foods) while it is 0.007% for the additive; for estragole (in spices), the natural occurrence HERP is 0.001% compared to 0.0002% for the additive; for methyleugenol, the natural occurrence (in spices) HERP is 0.004% compared to 0.0006% for the additive. For allyl isothiocyanate, the natural occurrence HERP in mustard is 0.0003% compared to 0.0002% for the additive; the natural value only includes mustard (Krul & al. 2002; Tsao & al. 2002) but allyl isothiocyanate is also present in other *Brassica* vegetables such as cabbage, cauliflower, and Brussels sprouts (Nijssen & al. 1996).

Safrole is the principle component (up to 90%) of oil of sassafras. It was formerly used as the main flavoring ingredient in root beer. It is also present in the oils of basil, nutmeg, and mace (Nijssen & al. 1996). The HERP value for average consumption of naturally occurring safrole in spices is 0.03%. Safrole and safrole-containing sassafras oils have been banned from use as food additives in the United States and Canada (Canada Gazette 1995; US Food and Drug Administration 1960). For a person consuming a glass of sassafras root beer per day for life (before the 1964 ban in the US), the HERP value would have been 0.2% (Ames & al. 1987). Sassafras root can still be purchased in health food stores and can, therefore, be used to make tea; the recipe is on the World Wide Web.

Butylated hydroxyanisole (BHA)

BHA is a phenolic antioxidant that is "Generally Regarded as Safe" (GRAS) by the FDA. By 1987, after BHA was shown to be a rodent carcinogen, its use declined six-fold (HERP = 0.002%) (US Food and Drug Administration 1991a); this was due to voluntary replacement by other antioxidants and to the fact that the use of animal fats and oils, in which BHA is primarily used as an antioxidant, has consistently declined in the United States. The mechanistic and carcinogenicity results on BHA indicate that malignant tumors were induced only at a dose above the MTD at which cell division was increased in the forestomach, which is the only site of tumorigenesis; the proliferation is only at high doses and is dependent on continuous dosing until late in the experiment (Clayson & al. 1990). Humans do not have a forestomach. We note that the dose-response for BHA curves sharply upward but the potency value used in HERP is based on a linear model; if the California EPA potency value (which is based on a linearized multistage model) were used in HERP instead of TD_{50}, the HERP values for BHA would be 25 times lower (California Environmental Protection Agency, Standards and Criteria Work Group 1994). A recent epidemiological study in the Netherlands found no association between BHA consumption and stomach cancer in humans (Botterweck & al. 2000).

Saccharin

Saccharin, which has largely been replaced by other sweeteners, has been shown to induce tumors in rodents by a mechanism that is not relevant to humans. Recently, both the NTP and the IARC re-evaluated the potential carcinogenic risk of saccharin to humans. NTP delisted saccharin in its *Report on Carcinogens* (US National Toxicology Program 2000b) and the IARC downgraded its evaluation to Group 3, "not classifiable as to carcinogenicity to humans" (International Agency for Research on Cancer

1999b). There is convincing evidence that the induction of bladder tumors in rats by sodium saccharin requires a high dose and is related to development of a calcium phosphate-containing precipitate in the urine (Cohen 1995), which is not relevant to human dietary exposures. In a 24-year study by the US National Cancer Institute (NCI), rhesus and cynomolgus monkeys were fed a dose of sodium saccharin that was equivalent to 5 cans of diet soda daily for 11 years (Thorgeirsson & al. 1994). The average daily dose-rate of sodium saccharin was about 100 times lower than the dose that was carcinogenic to rats (Gold & al. 1999; Gold & al. 1997c). There was no carcinogenic effect in monkeys. There was also no effect on the urine or urothelium, no evidence of increased urothelial-cell proliferation or of formation of solid material in the urine (Takayama & al. 1998). One would not expect to find a carcinogenic effect under the conditions of the monkey study because of the low dose administered (Gold & al. 1999). However, there may also be a true species difference because primate urine has a low concentration of protein and is less concentrated (lower osmolality) than rat urine (Takayama & al. 1998). Human urine is similar to monkey urine in this respect (Cohen 1995).

Mycotoxins
Of the 23 fungal toxins tested for carcinogenicity, 14 are positive (61%) (table 4). The mutagenic mold toxin, aflatoxin, which is found in moldy peanut and corn products, interacts with chronic hepatitis infection in the development of human liver cancer (Qian & al. 1994). There is a synergistic effect in the human liver between aflatoxin (genotoxic effect) and the hepatitis B virus (cell division effect) in the induction of liver cancer (Wu-Williams & al. 1992). The HERP value for aflatoxin of 0.008% is based on the rodent potency. If the lower human potency value calculated by FDA from epidemiological data were used instead, the HERP would be about 10-fold lower (US Food and Drug

Administration 1993a). Aflatoxin also induced liver tumors in cynomolgus and rhesus monkeys and the HERP value using TD_{50} in monkeys would be between the value for rodents and humans. Biomarker measurements of aflatoxin in populations in Africa and China, which have high rates of hepatitis B and C viruses and liver cancer, confirm that those populations are chronically exposed to high levels of aflatoxin (Groopman & al. 1992; Pons 1979). Liver cancer is unusual in the United States and Canada (about 2% of cancer deaths) and is more common among men than women (National Cancer Institute of Canada 2001; Ries & al. 2000). In the United States, an increase in liver cancer in the early 1990s was most likely due to the spread of hepatitis virus infection transmitted by transfusions (before screening of blood products for HCV), use of intravenous drugs, and sexual practices 10 to 30 years earlier (El-Serag & Mason 1999; Ince & Wands 1999). In the United States, one study estimated that hepatitis viruses can account for half of liver cancer cases among non-Asians and even more among Asians (Yu & al. 1991).

Ochratoxin A, a potent rodent carcinogen (Gold & Zeiger 1997), has been measured in Europe and Canada in agricultural and meat products. An estimated exposure of 1 ng/kg/day would have a HERP value at about the median of table 5 (International Life Sciences Institute February 1996; Kuiper-Goodman & Scott 1989).

The persistent contaminants, PCBs and TCDD
Polychlorinated biphenyls (PCBs) and tetrachlorodibenzo-*p*-dioxin (TCDD, dioxin), which have been a concern because of their environmental persistence and carcinogenic potency in rodents, are primarily consumed in foods of animal origin. In the United States, PCBs are no longer used but some exposure persists. Consumption in food in the United States declined about 20-fold between 1978 and 1986 (Gartrell & al. 1986; Gunderson 1995). PCBs, which are

not flammable, were formerly used as coolants and lubricants in electrical equipment. The HERP value for PCB in table 5 for the most recent reporting in the FDA Total Diet Study (1984–1986) is 0.00008%, towards the bottom of the ranking, and far below many values for naturally occurring chemicals in common foods. It has been reported that some countries may have higher intakes of PCBs than the United States (World Health Organization 1993). A recent epidemiological study, in which PCBs were measured in the blood of women on Long Island, found no association between PCBs and breast cancer (Gammon & al. 2002).

TCDD, the most potent rodent carcinogen, is produced naturally by burning when chloride ion is present, for example, in forest fires or wood burning in homes. The EPA (US Environmental Protection Agency 2000) estimates that the source of TCDD is primarily from the atmosphere directly from emissions (e.g. incinerators or burning trash), or indirectly by returning dioxin that is already in the environment to the atmosphere (US Environmental Protection Agency 1994a; U.S. Environmental Protection Agency 2001). TCDD bioaccumulates through the food chain because of its lipophilicity, and more than 95% of human intake is from animal fats in the diet (US Environmental Protection Agency 2001). Dioxin emissions decreased by 75% from 1987 to 1995, which EPA primarily attributes to reduced medical and municipal incineration emissions. The decline continues (US Environmental Protection Agency 2001). Estimates of dietary intake can vary because TCDD is often not detected in samples of animal products (about 60% of such samples have no detectable TCDD). Intake estimates are based on an assumption that dioxin is present in food at one-half the limit of detection when no dioxin is detected; the intake estimate would be lower by about half if zero were assumed instead (Schecter & al. 2001).

TCDD, which is not genotoxic (US Environmental Protection Agency 2000), exerts many of its harmful effects in experimental animals through binding to the *Ah receptor (AhR)*, and does not have effects in the *AhR knockout mouse* (Birnbaum 1994; Fernandez-Salguero & al. 1996). A wide variety of natural substances also bind to the Ah receptor (e.g., tryptophan oxidation products) and, insofar as they have been examined, they have similar properties to TCDD (Ames & al. 1990), including inhibition of estrogen-induced effects in rodents (Safe & al. 1998). For example, a variety of flavones and other plant substances in the diet and their metabolites bind to the receptor or are converted in the stomach to chemicals that bind to the Ah receptor; e.g. indole-3-carbinol (I3C). I3C is the main metabolite of glucobrassicin, a natural chemical that is present in large amounts in vegetables of the *Brassica* genus, including broccoli, and gives rise to the potent Ah binder, indole carbazole (Bradfield & Bjeldanes 1987). In comparing possible harmful effects, the binding affinity (greater for TCDD) and amounts in the diet (much greater for dietary compounds) both need to be considered. Some studies provide evidence that I3C enhances carcinogenicity (Dashwood 1998). Additionally, both I3C and TCDD, when administered to pregnant rats, resulted in reproductive abnormalities in male offspring (Wilker & al. 1996). Currently, I3C is in clinical trials for prevention of breast cancer (Kelloff & al. 1996a; Kelloff & al. 1996b; US National Toxicology Program 2000a) and is also being tested for carcinogenicity by the NTP (US National Toxicology Program 2000a). I3C is marketed as a dietary supplement at recommended doses about 30 times higher (Theranaturals 2000) than present in the average Western diet (US National Toxicology Program 2000a).

TCDD has received enormous scientific and regulatory attention, and controversy abounds about possible health risks to humans. It has been speculated that nearly 7000 publications have been written and US$3–5 billion has been spent to assess dioxin exposure and health effects to humans and wildlife (Paustenbach 2002, in press). The US EPA has been estimating dioxin cancer risk since 1991 (US Environmental Protection Agency 1994a; US Environmental Protection Agency 1994b; US Environmental Protection Agency 1995; US Environmental Protection Agency 2000), and the EPA Science Advisory Board has recently recommended reconsideration of many issues in the EPA assessment (Paustenbach 2002, in press; Science Advisory Board 2001). A committee of the US National Academy of Sciences has been appointed to evaluate the risks from dioxins in the diet.

The IARC evaluated TCDD as a human carcinogen (Group 1) on the basis of overall cancer mortality, even though no specific type of cancer was found to be increased in the epidemiological studies of formerly highly exposed workers (International Agency for Research on Cancer 1997). An IARC evaluation based on overall cancer mortality is unprecedented. With respect to risks, IARC concluded that:

> Evaluation of the relationship between the magnitude of the exposure in experimental systems and the magnitude of the response (i.e. dose-response relationships) do not permit conclusions to be drawn on the human health risks from background exposures to 2,3,7,8-TCDD. (International Agency for Research on Cancer 1997: 342)

The US NTP *Ninth Report on Carcinogens* concurred with IARC in the human carcinogen evaluation (US National Toxicology Program 2000b; US National Toxicology Program 2001). The EPA characterized TCDD as a "human carcinogen" but concluded that "there is no clear indication of increased disease in the general population attributable to dioxin-like compounds" (US Environmental Protection Agency 2000; US Environmental Protection Agency 2001). One meta-analysis combined the worker studies and found that there was no increasing cancer mortality, overall or for a specific organ, with increasing exposure to TCDD (Starr 2001). The most recent meta-analysis, using additional follow-up data, found an increased trend in total cancer mortality with increasing TCDD exposure (Crump & al. 2003, in press).

Worldwide, dioxin has primarily been regulated by many groups on the basis of sensitive reproductive and developmental (non-cancer) effects in experimental animals, which have a threshold. In contrast, the US EPA estimates have used cancer potency factors and a standard linear risk assessment model. The level of acceptable intake for humans has been judged similarly by many groups: the World Health Organization (Van den Berg & al. 1998), the US Agency for Toxic Substances and Disease Registry (ATSDR) (Agency for Toxic Substances and Disease Registry 1998), the European Community (European Commission Scientific Committee on Foods 2001), Health and Welfare Canada (Ministry of Environment and Energy 1997), and the Japanese Environmental Agency (Japanese Environmental Agency 1999). The acceptable level set by these groups differs from the US EPA assessments that are based on cancer: the risks levels that are considered to be safe are 1,000 to 10,000 times higher (less stringent) than the levels that the EPA draft documents would consider to be a negligible risk (one-in-a-million cancer risk). All of the agencies, including the US EPA, have based their evaluations on Toxic Equivalency (TEQ), a method that combines exposures to all dioxins and dioxin-like compounds. These agencies also take into consideration the body-burden doses of dioxins in humans due to bioaccumulation in lipid. There are uncertainties in these methods: for example, the TEQ method assumes that the toxic effects of many compounds are additive; however, antagonistic effects have been reported among these chemicals in experimental studies (European Commission Scientific Committee on Foods 2000). The EPA risk estimates thus provide a worst-case risk; actual risks are unlikely to be greater and may be substantially less. The EPA Science Advisory Board (SAB) has recommended reconsideration of many aspects of the EPA cancer risk assessment, including the classification as a known human carcinogen, methods to estimate cancer potency and noncancer effects, uncertainties in estimation of body burden of dioxins, and consideration of dose-response curves other than a linear one (Agency for Toxic Substances and Disease Registry 1998; Paustenbach 2002, in press; Science Advisory Board 2001).

In table 5, the HERP value of 0.0003%, which is for average US intake of TCDD, is below the median of the values in table 5. If the exposures to all dioxin-like compounds were used for the exposure estimate (TEQ), then the HERP value would be 10 times greater. If the body burden of these combined dioxins were also considered in HERP as the EPA has done, then the combined effect of these two factors would make the HERP value 30 times greater (HERP would be 0.01%), but would not be comparable to the other HERP values in table 5 because of combining exposures to several chemicals [TEQ] and considering exposure due to bioaccumulation).

Summary of HERP analysis

In sum, the HERP analysis in table 5 demonstrates the ubiquitous exposures to rodent carcinogens in everyday life and documents that possible hazards from the background of naturally occurring rodent carcinogens are present throughout the ranking. Widespread exposures to naturally occurring rodent carcinogens cast doubt on the relevance to human cancer of low-level exposures to synthetic rodent carcinogens. In regulatory efforts to prevent human cancer, the evaluation of low-level exposures to synthetic chemicals has had a high priority. Our results indicate, however, that a high percentage of both natural and synthetic chemicals are rodent carcinogens at the MTD and that tumor incidence data from rodent bioassays are not adequate to assess low-dose risk. Moreover, there is an imbalance in the testing of synthetic chemicals compared to that of natural chemicals. There is a background of natural chemicals in the diet that rank at or near the median HERP value, even though so few natural chemicals have been tested in rodent bioassays. In table 5, 90% of the HERP values are above the level that has been used for as the virtually safe dose (VSD) in regulatory policy for rodent carcinogens.

Caution is necessary in drawing conclusions from the occurrence in the diet of natural chemicals that are rodent carcinogens. It is not argued here that these dietary exposures are necessarily of much relevance to human cancer. The major known causes of human cancer are not single chemical agents like those studied in rodent bioassays (**Misconception 2, p. 7**).

Table 5: Ranking possible carcinogenic hazards from average US exposures to rodent carcinogens

Description of columns

The first column, **Possible hazard HERP (%)** is calculated using the information in columns 2, 3, and 4. The second column, **Average daily US (human) exposure**, indicates a daily dose for a lifetime from drugs, the air in the workplace or home, food, water, residues, etc. The third column, **Human dose of rodent carcinogen**, is divided by 70 kg to give a mg/kg/day of human exposure. The *Human Exposure/Rodent Potency index (HERP)* in column 1 expresses this human dose as a percentage of the *TD_{50}* in the rodent (mg/kg/day), which is reported in column 4, on the right-hand page of table 5. TD_{50} values used in the HERP calculation are averages calculated by taking the harmonic mean of the TD_{50}s of the positive tests in that species from the *Carcinogenic Potency Database*. Average TD_{50} values have been calculated separately for rats and mice, and the more potent value is used for calculating possible hazard. (See **Appendix**, p. 97, for more details.)

Table 5(1): Ranking possible carcinogenic hazards

Possible hazard HERP (%)	Average daily US (human) exposure (Chemicals that occur naturally in foods are in bold.)	Human dose of rodent carcinogen
140	EDB: production workers (high exposure) (before 1977)	Ethylene dibromide, 150 mg
17	Clofibrate	Clofibrate, 2 g
12	**Phenobarbital, 1 sleeping pill**	Phenobarbital, 60 mg
6.9	Gemfibrozil	Gemfibrozil, 1.2 g
6.8	Styrene-butadiene rubber industry workers (1978-86)	1,3-Butadiene, 66.0 mg
6.2	**Comfrey-pepsin tablets, 9 daily (no longer recommended)**	Comfrey root, 2.7 g
6.1	Tetrachloroethylene: dry cleaners with dry-to-dry units (1980-90)	Tetrachloroethylene, 433 mg
4.0	Formaldehyde: production workers (1979)	Formaldehyde, 6.1 mg
3.6	**Alcoholic beverages, all types**	Ethyl alcohol, 22.8 ml
2.4	Acrylonitrile: production workers (1960-1986)	Acrylonitrile, 28.4 mg
2.2	Trichloroethylene: vapor degreasing (before 1977)	Trichloroethylene, 1.02 g
1.8	**Beer, 229 g**	Ethyl alcohol, 11.7 ml
1.4	Mobile home air (14 hours/day)	Formaldehyde, 2.2 mg
1.3	**Comfrey-pepsin tablets, 9 daily (no longer recommended)**	Symphytine, 1.8 mg
0.9	Methylene chloride: workers, industry average (1940s-80s)	Methylene chloride, 471 mg

from average US exposures to rodent carcinogens

Potency TD$_{50}$ (mg/kg/day)[a]		Exposure references
Rats	Mice	
1.52	(7.45)	Ott & al. 1980; Ramsey & al. 1978
169	•	Havel & Kane 1982
(+)	7.38	American Medical Association Division of Drugs 1983
247	(–)	Arky 1998
(261)	13.9	Matanoski & al. 1993
626	•	Culvenor & al. 1980; Hirono & al. 1978
101	(126)	Andrasik & Cloutet 1990
2.19	(43.9)	Siegal & al. 1983
9110	(–)	Nephew & al. 2000
16.9	•	Blair & al. 1998
668	(1580)	Page & Arthur 1978
9110	(–)	Beer Institute 1999
2.19	(43.9)	Connor & al. 1985
1.91	•	Culvenor & al. 1980; Hirono & al. 1978
724	(1100)	CONSAD Research Corporation 1990

Table 5(2): Ranking possible carcinogenic hazards

Possible hazard HERP (%)	Average daily US (human) exposure	Human dose of rodent carcinogen
(Chemicals that occur naturally in foods are in bold.)		
0.6	Wine, 20.8 g	Ethyl alcohol, 3.67 ml
0.5	Dehydroepiandrosterone (DHEA)	DHEA supplement, 25 mg
0.4	Conventional home air (14 hours/day)	Formaldehyde, 598 µg
0.2	Fluvastatin	Fluvastatin, 20 mg
0.1	d-Limonene in food	d-Limonene, 15.5 mg
0.1	Coffee, 11.6 g	Caffeic acid, 20.8 mg
0.06	Lovastatin	Lovastatin, 20 mg
0.04	Lettuce, 14.9 g	Caffeic acid, 7.90 mg
0.03	Safrole in spices	Safrole, 1.2 mg
0.03	Orange juice, 138 g	d-Limonene, 4.28 mg
0.03	Comfrey herb tea, 1 cup (1.5 g root) (no longer recommended)	Symphytine, 38 µg
0.03	Tomato, 88.7 g	Caffeic acid, 5.46 mg
0.03	Furfural in food	Furfural, 3.64 mg
0.02	Coffee, 11.6 g	Catechol, 1.16 mg
0.02	Mushroom (*Agaricus bisporus* 2.55 g)	Mixture of hydrazines, etc. (whole mushroom)

from average US exposures to rodent carcinogens

Potency TD$_{50}$ (mg/kg/day)[a]		Exposure references
Rats	Mice	
9110	(–)	Wine Institute 2001
68.1	•	
2.19	(43.9)	McCann & al. 1987
125	•	Arky 1998
204	(–)	Stofberg & Grundschober 1987
297	(4900)	Clarke & Macrae 1988; Coffee Research Institute 2001
(–)	515	Arky 1998
297	(4900)	Herrmann 1978; Technical Assessment Systems 1989
(441)	51.3	Hall & al. 1989
204	(–)	Schreier & al. 1979; Technical Assessment Systems 1989
1.91	•	Culvenor & al. 1980
297	(4900)	Schmidtlein & Herrmann 1975a; Technical Assessment Systems 1989
(683)	197	Adams & al. 1997
84.7	(244)	Coffee Research Institute 2001; Rahn & König 1978; Tressl & al. 1978
(–)	20,300	Matsumoto & al. 1991; Stofberg & Grundschober 1987; Toth & Erickson 1986

Table 5(3): Ranking possible carcinogenic hazards

Possible hazard HERP (%)	Average daily US (human) exposure	Human dose of rodent carcinogen
(Chemicals that occur naturally in foods are in bold.)		
0.02	**Apple, 32.0 g**	Caffeic acid, 3.40 mg
0.01	BHA: daily US avg (1975)	BHA, 4.6 mg
0.01	**Beer (before 1979), 229 g**	Dimethylnitrosamine, 646 ng
0.008	Aflatoxin: daily US avg (1984–1989)	Aflatoxin, 18 ng
0.007	**Celery, 14 g**	Caffeic acid, 1.51 mg
0.007	d-Limonene	Food additive, 1.01 mg
0.007	**Cinnamon, 21.9 mg**	Coumarin, 65.0 µg
0.006	**Coffee, 11.6 g**	Furfural, 783 µg
0.005	**Coffee, 11.6 g**	Hydroquinone, 290 µg
0.005	Saccharin: daily US avg (1977)	Saccharin, 7 mg
0.005	**Carrot, 12.1 g**	Aniline, 624 µg
0.004	**Bread, 79 g**	Furfural, 584 µg
0.004	**Potato, 54.9 g**	Caffeic acid, 867 µg
0.004	Methyl eugenol in food	Methyl eugenol, 46.2 µg
0.003	Conventional home air (14 hour/day)	Benzene, 155 µg

from average US exposures to rodent carcinogens

Potency TD$_{50}$ (mg/kg/day)[a]		Exposure references
Rats	**Mice**	
297	(4900)	Mosel & Herrmann 1974; US Evironmental Protection Agency, Office of Pesticide Programs 1989
606	(5530)	US Food and Drug Administration 1991a
0.0959	(0.189)	Beer Institute 1999; Fazio & al. 1980; Preussmann & Eisenbrand 1984
0.0032	(+)	US Food and Drug Administration 1992
297	(4900)	Smiciklas-Wright & al. 2002; Stöhr & Herrmann 1975
204	(−)	Lucas & al. 1999
13.9	(103)	Poole & Poole 1994
(683)	197	Coffee Research Institute 2001; Stofberg & Grundschober 1987
82.8	(225)	Coffee Research Institute 2001; Heinrich & Baltes 1987; Tressl & al. 1978
2140	(−)	National Research Council 1979
194[b]	(−)	Neurath & al. 1977; Technical Assessment Systems 1989
(683)	197	Smiciklas-Wright & al. 2002; Stofberg & Grundschober 1987
297	(4900)	Schmidtlein & Herrmann 1975b; Technical Assessment Systems 1989
(19.7)	18.6	Smith & al. 2002
(169)	77.5	McCann & al. 1987

Table 5(4): Ranking possible carcinogenic hazards

Possible hazard HERP (%)	Average daily US (human) exposure	Human dose of rodent carcinogen
	(Chemicals that occur naturally in foods are in bold.)	
0.002	Coffee, 11.6 g	4-Methylcatechol, 378 µg
0.002	Nutmeg, 17.6 mg	d-Limonene, 299 µg
0.002	Carrot, 12.1 g	Caffeic acid, 374 µg
0.002	Ethylene thiourea: daily US avg (1990)	Ethylene thiourea, 9.51 µg
0.002	BHA: daily US avg (1987)	BHA, 700 µg
0.002	DDT: daily US avg (before 1972 ban)[5]	DDT, 13.8 µg
0.001	**Estragole in spices**	Estragole, 54.0 µg
0.001	**Pear, 3.7 g**	Caffeic acid, 270 µg
0.001	Toxaphene: daily US avg (before 1982 ban)[c]	Toxaphene, 6.43 µg
0.001	**Mushroom (*Agaricus bisporus* 5.34 g)**	Glutamyl-p-hydrazino-benzoate, 224 µg
0.001	**Plum, 1.7 g**	Caffeic acid, 235 µg
0.001	[UDMH: daily US avg (1988)]	[UDMH, 2.82 µg (from Alar)]
0.001	Bacon, 19 g	Diethylnitrosamine, 19 ng
0.0008	Bacon, 19 g	Dimethylnitrosamine, 57.0 ng

from average US exposures to rodent carcinogens

Potency TD$_{50}$ (mg/kg/day)[a]		Exposure references
Rats	**Mice**	
248	•	Coffee Research Institute 2001; Heinrich & Baltes 1987; International Agency for Research on Cancer 1991
204	(–)	Bejnarowicz & Kirch 1963; US Department of Agriculture 2000
297	(4900)	Stöhr & Herrmann 1975; Technical Assessment Systems 1989
7.9	(23.5)	US Environmental Protection Agency 1991a
606	(5530)	US Food and Drug Administration 1991a
(84.7)	12.8	Duggan & Corneliussen 1972
•	51.8	Smith & al. 2002
297	(4900)	Mosel & Herrmann 1974; US Environmental Protection Agency 1997
(–)	7.51	Podrebarac 1984
•	277	Chauhan & al. 1985; US Food and Drug Administration 2002
297	(4900)	Mosel & Herrmann 1974; US Environmental Protection Agency 1997
(–)	3.96	US Environmental Protection Agency, Office of Pesticide Programs 1989
0.0266	(+)	Sen & al. 1979; Smiciklas-Wright & al. 2002
0.0959	(0.189)	Smiciklas-Wright & al. 2002; Tricker & Preussmann 1991

Table 5(5): Ranking possible carcinogenic hazards

Possible hazard HERP (%)	Average daily US (human) exposure (Chemicals that occur naturally in foods are in bold.)	Human dose of rodent carcinogen
0.0008	Tap water, 1 liter (1987-92)	Chloroform, 51 µg
0.0008	DDE: daily US avg (before 1972 ban)c	DDE, 6.91 µg
0.0007	**Bacon, 19 g**	N-Nitrosopyrrolidine, 324 ng
0.0006	**Methyl eugenol**	Food additive, 7.7 µg
0.0004	EDB: Daily US avg (before 1984 ban)c	EDB, 420 ng
0.0004	Tap water, 1 liter (1987-92)	Bromodichloromethane, 13 µg
0.0004	**Celery, 14 g**	8-Methoxypsoralen, 8.56 µg
0.0003	**Mango, 1.0 g**	d-Limonene, 40.0 µg
0.0003	TCDD: daily US avg (1994)	TCDD, 5.4 pg
0.0003	Furfural	Food additive, 36.4 µg
0.0003	Carbaryl: daily US avg (1990)	Carbaryl, 2.6 µg
0.0003	**Mustard, 18.9 mg**	Allyl isothiocyanate, 17.4 µg
0.0002	**Beer (1994-95), 229 g**	Dimethylnitrosamine, 16 ng
0.0002	**Mushroom (*Agaricus bisporus*, 5.34 g)**	p-Hydrazinobenzoate, 58.6 µg
0.0002	Estragole	Food additive, 5.79 µg

from average US exposures to rodent carcinogens

Potency TD$_{50}$ (mg/kg/day)[a]		Exposure references
Rats	Mice	
(262)	90.3	American Water Works Association, Government Affairs Office 1993; McKone 1987; McKone 1993
(–)	12.5	Duggan & Corneliussen 1972
(0.799)	0.679	Stofberg & Grundschober 1987; Tricker & Preussmann 1991
(19.7)	18.6	Smith & al. 2002
1.52	(7.45)	US Environmental Protection Agency, Office of Pesticide Programs February 8, 1984
(72.5)	47.7	American Water Works Association. Government Affairs Office 1993
32.4	(–)	Beier & al. 1983; Smiciklas-Wright & al. 2002
204	(–)	Engel & Tressl 1983; US Environmental Protection Agency 1997
0.0000235	(0.000156)	US Environmental Protection Agency 2000
(683)	197	Lucas & al. 1999
14.1	(–)	US Food and Drug Administration 1991b
96	(–)	Krul & al. 2002; Lucas & al. 1999; Tsao & al. 2002
0.0959	(0.189)	Beer Institute 1999; Glória & al. 1997
•	454[b]	Chauhan & al. 1985; US Food and Drug Administration 2002
•	51.8	Lucas & al. 1999

Table 5(6): Ranking possible carcinogenic hazards

Possible hazard HERP (%)	Average daily US (human) exposure	Human dose of rodent carcinogen
	(Chemicals that occur naturally in foods are in bold.)	
0.0002	Allyl isothiocyanate	Food additive, 10.5 µg
0.0002	**Hamburger, pan fried, 85 g**	PhIP, 176 ng
0.0001	Toxaphene: daily US avg (1990)c	Toxaphene, 595 ng
0.00008	PCBs: daily US avg (1984-86)	PCBs, 98 ng
0.00008	**Toast, 79 g**	Urethane, 948 ng
0.00008	DDE/DDT: daily US avg (1990)c	DDE, 659 ng
0.00007	**Beer, 229 g**	Furfural, 9.50 µg
0.00006	**Parsnip, 48.8 mg**	8-Methoxypsoralen, 1.42 µg
0.00004	**Parsley, fresh, 257 mg**	8-Methoxypsoralen, 928 ng
0.00003	**Hamburger, pan fried, 85 g**	MeIQx, 38.1 ng
0.00002	Dicofol: daily US avg (1990)	Dicofol, 544 ng
0.00001	**Hamburger, pan fried, 85 g**	IQ, 6.38 ng
0.000009	**Beer, 229 g**	Urethane, 102 ng
0.000005	Hexachlorobenzene: daily US avg (1990)	Hexachlorobenzene, 14 ng
0.000001	Lindane: daily US avg (1990)	Lindane, 32 ng

from average US exposures to rodent carcinogens

Potency TD$_{50}$ (mg/kg/day)[a]		Exposure references
Rats	**Mice**	
96	(–)	Lucas & al. 1999
1.64[b]	(28.6)[b]	Knize & al. 1994; Technical Assessment Systems 1989
(–)	7.51	US Food and Drug Administration 1991b
1.74	(9.58)	Gunderson 1995
(41.3)	16.9	Canas & al. 1989; Smiciklas-Wright & al. 2002
(–)	12.5	US Food and Drug Administration 1991b
(683)	197	Beer Institute 1999; Lau & Lindsay 1972; Tressl 1976; Wheeler & al. 1971
32.4	(–)	Ivie & al. 1981; US Environmental Protection Agency 1997
32.4	(–)	Chaudhary & al. 1986; US Environmental Protection Agency 1997
1.66	(24.3)	Knize & al. 1994; Technical Assessment Systems 1989
(–)	32.9	US Food and Drug Administration 1991b
0.921[b]	(19.6)	Knize & al. 1994; Technical Assessment Systems 1989
(41.3)	16.9	Beer Institute 1999; Canas & al. 1989
3.86	(65.1)	US Food and Drug Administration 1991b
(–)	30.7	US Food and Drug Administration 1991b

Table 5(7): Ranking possible carcinogenic hazards

Possible hazard HERP (%)	Average daily US (human) exposure	Human dose of rodent carcinogen
	(Chemicals that occur naturally in foods are in bold.)	
0.0000004	PCNB: daily US avg (1990)	PCNB (Quintozene), 19.2 ng
0.0000001	Chlorobenzilate: daily US avg (1989)c	Chlorobenzilate, 6.4 ng
0.00000008	Captan: daily US avg (1990)	Captan, 115 ng
0.00000001	Folpet: daily US avg (1990)	Folpet, 12.8 ng
<0.00000001	Chlorothalonil: daily US avg (1990)	Chlorothalonil, <6.4 ng

Note a: • = no data in Carcinogenic Potency Database; a number in parentheses indicates a TD_{50} value not used in the HERP calculation because TD_{50} is less potent than in the other species; (–) = negative in cancer test(s); (+) = positive cancer test(s) not suitable for calculating a TD_{50}.

Note b: TD_{50} harmonic mean was estimated for the base chemical from the hydrochloride salt.

from average US exposures to rodent carcinogens

Potency TD$_{50}$ (mg/kg/day)[a]		Exposure references
Rats	Mice	
(–)	71.1	US Food and Drug Administration 1991b
(–)	93.9	US Food and Drug Administration 1991b
2080	(2110)	US Food and Drug Administration 1991b
(–)	1550	US Food and Drug Administration 1991b
828[d]	(–)	US Environmental Protection Agency 1987; US Food and Drug Administration 1991b

Note c: No longer contained in any registered pesticide product (USEPA, 1998).

Note d: Additional data from the EPA that is not in the CPDB were used to calculate this TD$_{50}$ harmonic mean.

Misconception 8—Pesticides and other synthetic chemicals are disrupting hormones

Synthetic hormone mimics such as organochlorine pesticides have become an environmental issue (Colborn & al. 1996), which was recently addressed by the National Academy of Sciences (National Research Council 1999). We discussed in Misconception 2 that hormonal factors are important in human cancer and that life-style factors can markedly change the levels of endogenous hormones. The trace exposures to estrogenic organochlorine residues are tiny compared to the normal dietary intake of naturally occurring endocrine-active chemicals in fruits and vegetables (Safe 1995; Safe 1997; Safe 2000). These low levels of human exposure seem toxicologically implausible as a significant cause of cancer or of reproductive abnormalities (Reinli & Block 1996; Safe 1995; Safe 1997; Safe 2000). Recent *epidemiological* studies have found no association between organochlorine pesticides and breast cancer, including one in which DDT, DDE, dieldrin, and chlordane were measured in blood of women on Long Island (Gammon & al. 2002). Synthetic hormone mimics have been proposed as a cause of declining sperm counts, even though it has not been shown that sperm counts are declining (Becker & Berhane 1997; Gyllenborg & al. 1999; Kolata 1996; National Research

Council 1999; Saidi & al. 1999; Swan & al. 1997). A recent analysis for the United States examined all available data on sperm counts and found that mean sperm concentrations were higher in New York than all other American cities (Saidi & al. 1999). When this geographic difference was taken into account, there was no significant change in sperm counts for the past 50 years (Saidi & al. 1999). Even if sperm counts were declining, there are many more likely causes, such as smoking and diet (**Misconception 2**, p. 7).

Some recent studies have compared estrogenic equivalents (EQ) of dietary intake of synthetic chemicals to phytoestrogens in the normal diet, by considering both the amount humans consume and estrogenic potency. Results support the idea that synthetic residues are orders of magnitude lower in EQ and are generally weaker in potency. One study used a series of in vitro assays and calculated the EQs in extracts from 200 ml of Cabernet Sauvignon wine and the EQs from average intake of organochlorine pesticides (Gaido & al. 1998). EQs for a single glass of wine ranged from 0.15 to 3.68 µg/day compared to 1.24 ng/day for organochlorine pesticides (Gaido & al. 1998); thus, the organochlorine residues are roughly 1,000 times less.

Another study (Setchell & al. 1997) compared plasma concentrations of the phytoestrogens genistein and daidzein in infants fed soy-based formula rather than cow's milk formula or human breast milk. Mean plasma levels were hundreds of times higher for the soy-fed infants than for the others. Recent studies in mice suggest that genistein injected subcutaneously for 5 days early in life is carcinogenic; uterine adenocarcinomas were induced in mice at doses about 10-fold greater (mg/kg/day) than would be received by an infant who was fed on soy formula (Newbold & al. 2001).

Misconception 9—Regulation of low, hypothetical risks is effective in advancing public health

Since there is no risk-free world and resources are limited, society must set priorities in order to save the greatest number of lives (Graham & Wiener 1995; Hahn 1996). The EPA drew attention to the rising and sizeable cost to society of environmental regulations in its 1991 report *Environmental Investments: The Cost of a Clean Environment* (US Environmental Protection Agency 1991b). The EPA estimated that public and private costs in 1997 would be about $140 billion per year (about 2.6% of Gross National Product) (US Environmental Protection Agency 1991b).

Several economic analyses have concluded that current expenditures are not cost effective (Hahn & Stavins 2001); resources are not being used so as to save the greatest number of lives per dollar. One estimate is that the United States could prevent 60,000 deaths per year by redirecting the same dollar resources to more cost-effective programs (Tengs & al. 1995). For example, the median toxin control program costs 146 times more per life-year saved than the median medical intervention (Tengs & al. 1995). This difference is likely to be even greater because cancer risk estimates for toxin control programs are worst-case, hypothetical estimates, and the true risks at low dose are often likely to be zero (Gaylor & Gold 1995; Gold & al. 1998; Gold & al. 1992; **Misconception 5**). Some economists have argued that costly regulations intended to save lives may actually increase the number of deaths (Keeney 1990), in part because they divert resources from important health risks and in part because higher incomes are associated with lower mortality (Viscusi 1992; Wildavsky 1988; Wildavsky 1995). Rules on air and water pollution can be beneficial to health—it was a public-health benefit to phase lead out of gasoline—and clearly cancer prevention is not the only reason for regulations. However, worst-case assumptions in risk assessment represent a policy decision, not a scientific one, and they confuse attempts to allocate money effectively for risk abatement.

Regulatory efforts to reduce low-level human exposure to synthetic chemicals because they are rodent carcinogens are expensive since they aim to eliminate minuscule concentrations that can now be measured with improved techniques. These efforts distract from the major task of improving public health through increasing scientific understanding about how to prevent cancer (e.g., the role of diet), increasing public understanding of how life-style influences health, and improving our ability to help individuals alter life-style.

Glossary

Ah receptor (AhR): Aryl hydrocarbon receptor, a protein receptor in cells that binds dioxins at low concentration and mediates dioxin toxicity.

carcinogenic potency: An estimate of the lifetime daily dose-rate of a chemical that will give tumors to a specified percentage of animals in a cancer test. (See TD_{50}, LTD_{10}, and q_1^* for three measures of carcinogenic potency.)

Carcinogenic Potency Database (CPDB): A widely used and easily accessible resource on the standardized results of chronic, long-term animal cancer tests. See http://potency.berkeley.edu. Analyses are presented of 5,152 experiments on 1,298 chemicals reported in the published literature and include results sufficient for many investigations into carcinogenesis.

case-control study: An epidemiological study design in which individuals are selected based on the presence (case) or absence (control) of disease. Well-designed case-control studies require that the two groups be derived from the same population.

Chinese herb nephropathy: Kidney disease associated with consumption of the medicinal herb *aristolochia*.

chronic bioassay: An experiment to investigate the effects of a substance when administered chronically for life at the maximum dose that is predicted to be tolerated by test animals for a lifetime.

cohort study: An epidemiological study design in which individuals with known characteristics (occupational exposure, smoking, exercise, etc.) are enrolled and followed over time for specific outcomes. The rate of cancer (or other disease) in the exposed is compared to that in the unexposed. Relative rates of disease in people exposed to the variable of interest (e.g. fruit and vegetable consumption) are compared to the unexposed or the less exposed.

confounding factor: Confounding occurs because behavior-related variables of interest tend to cluster. An exposure (e.g., vegetable consumption) may be of interest in protecting against a particular cancer. However, if smokers eat fewer vegetables than non-smokers (they do), we may falsely attribute a risk reduction to vegetables that is really due to the fact that a higher proportion of vegetable eaters are non-smokers. Smoking, here, is a confounder of the association between vegetables and cancer. It can be controlled for by separating the smokers and the non-smokers and asking whether the vegetable-cancer association is seen in both groups (or by more sophisticated, but conceptually similar, statistical techniques).

CPDB: See Carcinogenic Potency Database

deficiency: Defined here as the dietary intake of a vitamin or mineral at a level <50% of the RDA, as distinguished from acute deficiency such as acute vitamin-C deficiency causing scurvy.

epidemiology: The study of patterns and causes of human health outcomes in a specified population.

HERP: An index of possible cancer hazard (Human Exposure/Rodent Potency, reported as a percent), which compares the dose of chemical to which humans are exposed vs. the estimate of the dose that gives tumors to half of test animals in a lifetime experiment.

inducibility: Ability to cause the synthesis of.

IQ: (2-amino-3-methylimidazo[4,5-*f*]quinoline), a mutagenic chemical formed naturally when meat, chicken, or fish is cooked at high temperatures. This heterocyclic amine is carcinogenic in rodent and monkey experiments.

LTD_{10}: The lower 95% confidence limit on the dose estimated to produce an extra lifetime cancer risk of 10% in an animal cancer test.

MeIQx: (2-amino-3,8-dimethylimidazo[4,5-*f*]quinoxaline), a mutagenic chemical formed naturally when meat, chicken, or fish is cooked at high temperatures. This heterocyclic amine is carcinogenic in rodent experiments.

mitochondria: The organelles in all cells that produce chemical energy (ATP) by removing electrons (burning or oxidizing) from fat or carbohydrate fuel and adding the electrons to oxygen.

NCI: United States National Cancer Institute

NTP: United States National Toxicology Program

oxidative damage: Damage from oxidants.

oxidative DNA lesions: Damage products in DNA from oxidants.

oxidative mutagens: Agents damaging DNA by removing electrons.

oxidative stress: Toxicity due to oxidants.

PDR: *Physician's Desk Reference*, the standard reference in the United States for prescription drugs.

PhIP: (2-amino-1-methyl-6-phenylimidazo[4,5-*b*]-pyridine), a mutagenic chemical formed naturally when meat, chicken, or fish is cooked at high temperatures; this heterocyclic amine is carcinogenic in rodent experiments.

q_i^*: The measure used by the US EPA for carcinogenic potency of a substance in an animal cancer test; a plausible 95% upper-bound estimate of the probability of cancer during a lifetime per unit dose.

recall bias: This can occur if individuals are describing events (exposures, diseases, pregnancy outcome, etc.) in the past in a non-comparable manner. It is primarily a problem in case-control studies when the presence of the disease in one group (cases) may result in differential recall (e.g. of alcohol consumption or dietary behavior) from that of controls.

TD_{50}: If there are no tumors in control animals, then TD_{50} is that chronic dose-rate in mg/kg body wt/day that would induce tumors in half the test animals at the end of a standard lifespan for the species. The average daily dose-rate estimated to halve the probability of remaining tumor-free throughout a lifespan experiment in test animals. The measure of carcinogenic potency in the CPDB.

TDS: The Total Diet Study of the United States Food and Drug Administration, which provides estimates of the total consumption of pesticide residues and other chemicals via food for specified age and gender groups. Conducted annually for more than 20 years.

Appendix—Method for calculating the HERP index

The HERP index takes into account both human exposures and the carcinogenic dose to rodents and compares them. HERP values indicate what percentage of the rodent carcinogenic daily dose (mg/kg/day) for 50% of test animals that a person receives from an average daily exposure (mg/kg/day).

For example, methyleugenol is a chemical that is carcinogenic in rats and mice and has a HERP value of 0.004% for average daily US exposure in food from its natural occurrence, and 0.0006% for average daily US exposure as a synthetic food additive. Below is an example of the HERP calculation for methyleugenol that occurs naturally (see table 5 at HERP = 0.004%). Data are available indicating that average naturally occurring methyleugenol consumption in the US is 46.2 µg/day (Smith & al. 2002). The calculation of HERP from the values in table 5 for methyleugenol is as follows:

(1) Human dose of rodent carcinogen is:
46.2 µg/day / 70 kg body weight = 0.66 µg/kg/day
(=0.00066 mg/kg/day);

(2) Rodent potency: the TD_{50} is 18.6 mg/kg/day in mice;

(3) Possible hazard (HERP) is:

$$\frac{0.0006 \text{ mg/kg/day human exposure}}{18.6 \text{ mg/kg/day TD}_{50}} = 0.00004; \ 0.00004 \times 100 = 0.004\%.$$

The TD_{50} values used in HERP are averages for rats and mice separately, calculated by taking the harmonic mean of the TD_{50} values from positive experiments. For methyleugenol, the TD_{50} in rats is 19.7 mg/kg/day and in mice 18.6 mg/kg/day. Since the mouse TD_{50} is lower (more potent), this value is used in HERP. Experiments in the CPDB that do not show an increase in tumors are ignored in HERP.

The TD_{50} value for rats or mice in the HERP table is a harmonic mean of the most potent TD_{50} values from each positive experiment.

The harmonic mean (T_H) is defined as:

$$T_H = \frac{1}{\dfrac{1}{n} \sum_{i=1}^{n} \dfrac{1}{T_i}}$$

References and further reading

Adachi, Y., Moore, L.E., Bradford, B.U., Gao, W., and Thurman, R.G. (1995). Antibiotics prevent liver injury in rats following long-term exposure to ethanol. *Gastroenterology* 108, 218–224.

Adams, T.B., Doull, J., Goodman, J.I., Munro, I.C., Newberne, P., Portoghese, P.S., Smith, R.L., Wagner, B.M., Weil, C.S., Woods, L.A., and Ford, R.A. (1997). The FEMA GRAS assessment of furfural used as a flavour ingredient. *Food Chem. Toxicol.* 35, 739–751.

Adamson, R.H., Takayama, S., Sugimura, T., and Thorgeirsson, U.P. (1994). Induction of hepatocellular carcinoma in nonhuman primates by the food mutagen 2-amino-3-methylimidazo[4,5-f]quinoline. *Environ. Health Perspect.* 102, 190–193.

Agency for Toxic Substances and Disease Registry (1998). *Toxicological profile for chlorinated dibenzo-p-dioxins (CDDs).* Centers for Disease Control, Atlanta, GA.

American Cancer Society (2000). *Cancer Facts & Figures—2000.* American Cancer Society, Atlanta, GA.

American Medical Association Division of Drugs (1983). *AMA Drug Evaluations.* AMA, Chicago, IL.

American Water Works Association, Government Affairs Office (1993). *Disinfectant/Disinfection By-Products Database for the Negotiated Regulation.* AWWA, Washington, DC.

Ames, B.N. (1998). Micronutrients prevent cancer and delay aging. *Toxicol. Lett.* 103, 5–18.

Ames, B.N., and Gold, L.S. (1989). Letter: Pesticides, risk, and applesauce. *Science* 244, 755–757. Letter: 244: 755.

Ames, B.N., and Gold, L.S. (1990). Chemical carcinogenesis: Too many rodent carcinogens. *Proc. Natl. Acad. Sci. USA* 87, 7772–7776. http://socrates.berkeley.edu/mutagen/PNAS1.html.

Ames, B.N., and Gold, L.S. (1991). Risk assessment of pesticides. *Chem. Eng. News* 69, 28–32, 48–49. Forum: pp. 27–55.

Ames, B.N., Gold, L.S., and Shigenaga, M.K. (1996). Cancer prevention, rodent high-dose cancer tests, and risk assessment. *Risk Anal.* 16, 613–617. http://potency.berkeley.edu/text/riskanaleditorial.html.

Ames, B.N., Gold, L.S., and Willett, W.C. (1995). The causes and prevention of cancer. *Proc. Natl. Acad. Sci. USA* 92, 5258–5265. http://socrates.berkeley.edu/mutagen/ames.pnas3.html.

Ames, B.N., Magaw, R., and Gold, L.S. (1987). Ranking possible carcinogenic hazards. *Science* 236, 271–280. Letters: 237: 235 (1987); 237: 1283–1284 (1987); 237: 1399–1400 (1987); 238: 1633–1634 (1987); Technical comment: 240: 1043–1047 (1988).

Ames, B.N., Motchnik, P.A., Fraga, C.G., Shigenaga, M.K., Hagen, T.M., and Ohlshan, A. (1994). Antioxidant prevention of birth defects and cancer. In *Male-Mediated Developmental Toxicity* (D.R. Mattison, ed.), pp. 243–259. Plenum Press, New York.

Ames, B.N., Profet, M., and Gold, L.S. (1990a). Dietary pesticides (99.99% all natural). *Proc. Natl. Acad. Sci. USA* 87, 7777–7781. http://socrates.berkeley.edu/mutagen/PNAS2.html.

Ames, B.N., Profet, M., and Gold, L.S. (1990b). Nature's chemicals and synthetic chemicals: Comparative toxicology. *Proc. Natl. Acad. Sci. USA* 87, 7782–7786.

Ames, B.N., Shigenaga, M.K., and Gold, L.S. (1993a). DNA lesions, inducible DNA repair, and cell division: Three key factors in mutagenesis and carcinogenesis. Environ. *Health Perspect.* 101 (Suppl. 5), 35–44.

Ames, B.N., Shigenaga, M.K., and Hagen, T.M. (1993b). Oxidants, antioxidants, and the degenerative diseases of aging. *Proc. Natl. Acad. Sci. USA* 90, 7915–7922.

Ames, B.N., and Wakimoto, P. (2002). Are vitamin and mineral deficiencies a major cancer risk? *Nature Rev. Cancer* 2, 694–704.

Anderson, R.N. (1999). United States life tables, 1997. *Natl. Vital Stat. Rep.* 47, 1–37.

Andrasik, J., and Cloutet, D. (1990). Monitoring solvent vapors in drycleaning plants. *Int. Fabricare Inst. Focus Dry Cleaning* 14, 1–8.

Arky, R. (1998). *Physicians' Desk Reference.* Medical Economics Company, Montvale, NJ.

Armstrong, B., and Doll, R. (1975). Environmental factors and cancer incidence and mortality in different countries, with special reference to dietary practices. *Int. J. Cancer* 15, 617–631.

Bailar, I., III, and Gornik, H.L. (1997). Cancer undefeated. *N. Engl. J. Med.* 336, 1569–1574.

Bailey, L.B., Wagner, P.A., Christakis, G.J., Araujo, P.E., Appledorf, H., Davis, C.G., Masteryanni, J., and Dinning, J.S. (1979). Folacin and iron status and hematological findings in predominately black elderly persons from urban low-income households. *Am. J. Clin. Nutr.* 32, 2346–2353.

Bailey, L.B., Wagner, P.A., Christakis, G.J., Davis, C.G., Appledorf, H., Araujo, P.E., Dorsey, E., and Dinning, J.S. (1982). Folacin and iron status and hematological findings in black and Spanish-American adolescents from urban low-income households. *Am. J. Clin. Nutr.* 35, 1023–1032.

Becker, S., and Berhane, K. (1997). A meta-analysis of 61 sperm count studies revisited. *Fertil. Steril.* 67, 1103–1108.

Beckman, K.B., and Ames, B.N. (1998). The free radical theory of aging matures. *Physiol. Rev.* 78, 547–581.

Beer Institute (1999). *1999 Brewers Almanac.* Beer Institute, Washington, DC. http://www.beerinstitute.org/pdfs/1999_Brewers_Almanac.pdf.

Beier, R.C., Ivie, G.W., Oertli, E.H., and Holt, D.L. (1983). HPLC analysis of linear furocoumarins (psoralens) in healthy celery *Apium graveolens. Food Chem. Toxicol.* 21, 163–165.

Bejnarowicz, E.A., and Kirch, E.R. (1963). Gas chromatographic analysis of oil of nutmeg. *J. Pharm. Sci.* 52, 988–993.

Berkley, S.F., Hightower, A.W., Beier, R.C., Fleming, D.W., Brokopp, C.D., Ivie, G.W., and Broome, C.V. (1986). Dermatitis in grocery workers associated with high natural concentrations of furanocoumarins in celery. *Ann Intern Med* 105, 351–355.

Bernstein, L., Gold, L.S., Ames, B.N., Pike, M.C., and Hoel, D.G. (1985). Some tautologous aspects of the comparison of carcinogenic potency in rats and mice. *Fundam. Appl. Toxicol.* 5, 79–86.

Bernstein, L., Henderson, B.E., Hanisch, R., Sullivan-Halley, J., and Ross, R.K. (1994). Physical exercise and reduced risk of breast cancer in young women. *J. Natl. Cancer Inst.* 86, 1403–1408.

Bernstein, L., Ross, R.K., and Pike, M.C. (1990). Hormone levels in older women; a study of postmenopausal breast cancer patients and healthy population controls. *Br. J. Cancer* 61, 298–302.

Birnbaum, L.S. (1994). The mechanism of dioxin toxicity: Relationship to risk assessment. *Environ. Health Perspect.* 102 (Suppl. 9), 157–167.

Bjerre, L.M., and LeLorier, J. (2001). Do statins cause cancer? A meta-analysis of large randomized clinical trials. *Am. J. Med.* 110, 716–723.

Blair, A., Stewart, P.A., Zaebst, D.D., Pottern, L., Zey, J.N., Bloom, T.F., Miller, B., Ward, E., and Lubin, J. (1998). Mortality of industrial workers exposed to acrylonitrile. *Scand. J. Work Environ. Health* 24 (Suppl. 2), 25–41.

Block, G. (1995). Are clinical trials really the answer? *Am. J. Clin. Nutr.* 62 (Suppl. 6), 1517–1520.

Block, G., Patterson, B., and Subar, A. (1992). Fruit, vegetables and cancer prevention: A review of the epidemiologic evidence. *Nutr. Cancer* 18, 1–29.

Block, G., Sinha, R., and Gridley, G. (1994). Collection of dietary-supplement data and implications for analysis. *Am. J. Clin. Nutr.* 59 (Suppl. 1), 232–239.

Blount, B.C., Mack, M.M., Wehr, C.M., MacGregor, J.T., Hiatt, R.A., Wang, G., Wickramasinghe, S.N., Everson, R.B., and Ames, B.N. (1997). Folate deficiency causes uracil misincorporation into human DNA and chromosome breakage: Implications for cancer and neuronal damage. *Proc. Natl. Acad. Sci. USA* 94, 3290–3295.

Bogen, K.T., and Gold, L.S. (1997). Trichloroethylene cancer risk: Simplified calculation of PBPK-based MCLs for cytotoxic endpoints. *Regul. Toxicol. Pharmacol.* 25, 26–42. http://www.idealibrary.com/links/doi/10.1006/rtph.1996.1070/pdf.

Bogen, K.T., and Keating, G.A. (2001). US dietary exposures to heterocyclic amines. *J. Expos. Anal. Environ. Epidem.* 11, 155–168.

Botterweck, A.A., van den Brandt, P.A., and Goldbohm, R.A. (1998). A prospective cohort study on vegetable and fruit consumption and stomach cancer risk in The Netherlands. *Am. J. Epidemiol.* 148, 842–853.

Botterweck, A.A.M., Verhagen, H., Goldbohm, R.A., Kleinjans, J., and van den Brandt, P.A. (2000). Intake of butylated hydroxyanisole and butylated hydroxytoluene and stomach cancer risk: Results from analyses in the Netherlands cohort study. *Food Chem. Toxicol.* 38, 599–605.

Boushey, C.J., Beresford, S.A., Omenn, G.S., and Motulsky, A.G. (1995). A quantitative assessment of plasma homocysteine as a risk factor for vascular disease. Probable benefits of increasing folic acid intakes. *J. Am. Med. Assoc.* 274, 1049–1057.

Bradfield, C.A., and Bjeldanes, L.F. (1987). Structure-activity relationships of dietary indoles: A proposed mechanism of action as modifiers of xenobiotic metabolism. *J. Toxicol. Environ. Health* 21, 311–323.

Burdock, G.A. (2000). Dietary supplements and lessons to be learned from GRAS. *Regul. Toxicol. Pharmacol.* 31, 68–76.

Butterworth, B.E., and Bogdanffy, M.S. (1999). A comprehensive approach for integration of toxicity and cancer risk assessments. *Regul. Toxicol. Pharmacol.* 29, 23–36.

Butterworth, B.E., Conolly, R.B., and Morgan, K.T. (1995). A strategy for establishing mode of action of chemical carcinogens as a guide for approaches to risk assessments. *Cancer Lett.* 93, 129–146.

Caan, B.J., Coates, A.O., Slattery, M.L., Potter, J.D., Quesenberry, C.P., Jr, and Edwards, S.M. (1998). Body size and the risk of colon cancer in a large case-control study. *Int. J. Obes. Relat. Metab. Disord.* 22, 178–184.

Calabrese, E.J., and Baldwin, L.A. (2001). Hormesis: A generalizable and unifying hypothesis. *Crit. Rev. Toxicol.* 31, 353–424.

California Department of Health Services (1985). *EDB Criteria Document.* CDHS, Sacramento, CA.

California Environmental Protection Agency. Standards and Criteria Work Group (1994). *California Cancer Potency Factors: Update.* CalEPA, Sacramento.

Canada Gazette (1995). The Food and Drugs Act.

Canas, B.J., Havery, D.C., Robinson, L.R., Sullivan, M.P., Joe, F.L., Jr., and Diachenko, G.W. (1989). Chemical contaminants monitoring: Ethyl carbamate levels in selected fermented foods and beverages. *J. Assoc. Off. Anal. Chem.* 72, 873–876.

Cattley, R.C., Illingworth, D.R., Laws, A., Pahor, M., Tobert, J.A., Newman, T.B., and Hulley, S.B. (1996). Carcinogenicity of lipid-lowering drugs (letters). *JAMA* 275, 1479–1482.

Chaudhary, S.K., Ceska, O., Tétu, C., Warrington, P.J., Ashwood-Smith, M.J., and Poulton, G.A. (1986). Oxypeucedanin, a major furocoumarin in parsley, *Petroselinum crispum*. *Planta Med.* 6, 462–464.

Chauhan, Y., Nagel, D., Gross, M., Cerny, R., and Toth, B. (1985). Isolation of N_2-[γ-L-(+)-glutamyl]-4-carboxyphenylhydrazine in the cultivated mushroom *Agaricus bisporus*. *J. Agric. Food Chem.* 33, 817–820.

Childs, M., and Girardot, G. (1992). Bilan des données acquises sur le risque à long terme des traitements hypolipidémiants. *Arch. Mal. Coeur Vaiss.* 85 (Spec. No. 2), 129–133.

Christen, S., Hagen, T.M., Shigenaga, M.K., and Ames, B.N. (1999). Chronic inflammation, mutation, and cancer. In *Microbes and Malignancy: Infection as a Cause of Cancer* (J. Parsonnet, ed.), pp. 35–88. Oxford University Press, New York.

Christensen, J.G., Goldsworthy, T.L., and Cattley, R.C. (1999). Dysregulation of apoptosis by c-myc in transgenic hepatocytes and effects of growth factors and nongenotoxic carcinogens. *Mol. Carcinog.* 25, 273–284.

Clarke, R.J., and Macrae, R., eds. (1988). *Coffee*. Elsevier, New York.

Clayson, D.B., and Iverson, F. (1996). Cancer risk assessment at the crossroads: The need to turn to a biological approach. *Regul. Toxicol. Pharmacol.* 24, 45–59.

Clayson, D.B., Iverson, F., Nera, E.A., and Lok, E. (1990). The significance of induced forestomach tumors. *Annu. Rev. Pharmacol. Toxicol.* 30, 441–463.

Coffee Research Institute (2001). *Consumption in the United States, Vol. 2002*. Coffee Research Institute. http://www.coffeeresearch.org/market/usa.htm.

Cohen, S.M. (1995). Role of urinary physiology and chemistry in bladder carcinogenesis. *Food Chem. Toxicol.* 33, 715–730.

Cohen, S.M. (1998). Cell proliferation and carcinogenesis. *Drug Metab. Rev.* 30, 339–357.

Cohen, S.M., and Lawson, T.A. (1995). Rodent bladder tumors do not always predict for humans. *Cancer Lett.* 93, 9–16.

Colborn, T., Dumanoski, D., and Myers, J.P. (1996). *Our Stolen Future: Are We Threatening Our Fertility, Intelligence, and Survival? A Scientific Detective Story*. Dutton, NY. http://www.osf-facts.org/.

Collins, J.J., Swaen, G.M., Marsh, G.M., Utidjian, H.M., Caporossi, J.C., and Lucas, L.J. (1989). Mortality patterns among workers exposed to acrylamide. *J. Occup. Med.* 31, 614–617.

Connor, T.H., Theiss, J.C., Hanna, H.A., Monteith, D.K., and Matney, T.S. (1985). Genotoxicity of organic chemicals frequently found in the air of mobile homes. *Toxicol. Letters* 25, 33–40.

CONSAD Research Corporation (1990). Final report. Economic analysis of OSHA's proposed standards for methylene chloride. OSHA Docket H-71.

Contrera, J., Jacobs, A., and DeGeorge, J. (1997). Carcinogenicity testing and the evaluation of regulatory requirements for pharmaceuticals. *Regul. Toxicol. Pharmacol.* 25, 130–145.

Crump, K.S., Canady, R., and Kogevinas, M. (2003, in press). Meta-analysis of dioxin cancer dose-response for three occupational cohorts. *Environmental Health Perspectives*.

Culvenor, C.C.J., Clarke, M., Edgar, J.A., Frahn, J.L., Jago, M.V., Peterson, J.E., and Smith, L.W. (1980). Structure and toxicity of the alkaloids of Russian comfrey (*Symphytum x Uplandicum nyman*), a medicinal herb and item of human diet. *Expcricntia* 36, 377–379.

Cunningham, M.L., Elwell, M.R., and Matthews, H.B. (1994a).

Relationship of carcinogenicity and cellular proliferation induced by mutagenic noncarcinogens vs carcinogens. III. Organophosphate pesticides vs. tris(2,3-dibromopropyl)phosphate. *Fundam. Appl. Toxicol.* 23, 363–369.

Cunningham, M.L., Foley, J., Maronpot, R.R., and Matthews, H.B. (1991). Correlation of hepatocellular proliferation with hepatocarcinogenicity induced by the mutagenic noncarcinogen:carcinogen pair—2,6- and 2,4-diaminotoluene. *Toxicol. Appl. Pharmacol.* 107, 562–567.

Cunningham, M.L., Maronpot, R.R., Thompson, M., and Bucher, J.R. (1994b). Early responses of the liver of B6C3F$_1$ mice to the hepatocarcinogen oxazepam. *Toxicol. Appl. Pharmacol.* 124, 31–38.

Czaja, M.J., Xu, J., Ju, Y., Alt, E., and Schmiedeberg, P. (1994). Lipopolysaccharide-neutralizing antibody reduces hepatocyte injury from acute hepatotoxin administration. *Hepatology* 19, 1282–1289.

Das, U.N. (2001). Is obesity an inflammatory condition? *Nutrition* 17, 953–966.

Dashwood, R.H. (1998). Indole-3-carbinol: Anticarcinogen or tumor promoter in *Brassica* vegetables? *Chem.-Biol. Interact.* 110, 1–5.

Davies, T.S., and Monro, A. (1995). Marketed human pharmaceuticals reported to be tumorigenic in rodents. *J. Am. Coll. Toxicol.* 14, 90–107.

Devesa, S.S., Blot, W.J., Stone, B.J., Miller, B.A., Tarone, R.E., and Fraumeni, F.J., Jr. (1995). Recent cancer trends in the United States. *J. Natl. Cancer Inst.* 87, 175–182.

Dich, J., Zahm, S.H., Hanberg, A., and Adami, H.-O. (1997). Pesticides and cancer. *Cancer Causes Control* 8, 420–443.

Doll, R., and Peto, R. (1981). *The Causes of Cancer.* Oxford University Press, New York.

Duggan, R.E., and Corneliussen, P.E. (1972). Dietary intake of pesticide chemicals in the United States (III), June 1968–April 1970. *Pest. Monit. J.* 5, 331–341.

El-Serag, H.B., and Mason, A.C. (1999). Rising incidence of hepatocellular carcinoma in the United States. *N. Engl. J. Med.* 340, 745–750.

Engel, K.H., and Tressl, R. (1983). Studies on the volatile components of two mango varieties. *J. Agric. Food Chem.* 31, 796–801.

European Commission Scientific Committee on Foods (2000). *Opinion of the SCF on the Risk Assessment of Dioxins and Dioxin-like PCBs in Food.* European Commisssion, Brussels, Belgium.

European Commission Scientific Committee on Foods (2001). *Opinion of the Scientific Committee on Food on the Risk Assessment of Dioxins and Dioxin-like PCBs in Food. Update Based on New Scientific Information Available Since the Adoption of the SCF Opinion of 22nd November 2000.* European Commisssion, Brussels, Belgium.

Fazio, T., Havery, D.C., and Howard, J.W. (1980). Determination of volatile N-nitrosamines in foodstuffs: I. A new clean-up technique for confirmation by GLC-MS. II. A continued survey of foods and beverages. In *N-Nitroso Compounds: Analysis, Formation and Occurrence* (E.A. Walker, L. Griciute, M. Castegnaro and M. Borzsonyi, eds.), Vol. 31, pp. 419–435. International Agency for Research on Cancer, Lyon, France.

Fenech, M., Aitken, C., and Rinaldi, J. (1998). Folate, vitamin B_{12}, homocysteine status and DNA damage in young Australian adults. *Carcinogenesis* 19, 1163–1171.

Fernandez-Salguero, P.M., Hilbert, D.M., Rudikoff, S., Ward, J.M., and Gonzalez, F.J. (1996). Aryl-hydrocarbon receptor-deficient mice are resistant to 2,3,7,8-tetrachlorodibenzo-*p*-dioxin-induced toxicity. *Toxicol. Appl. Pharmacol.* 140, 173–179.

Fraga, C.G., Motchnik, P.A., Shigenaga, M.K., Helbrook, H.J., Jacob, R.A., and Ames, B.N. (1991). Ascorbic acid protects against endogenous oxidative damage in human sperm. *Proc. Natl. Acad. Sci. USA* 88, 11003–11006.

Fraga, C.G., Motchnik, P.A., Wyrobek, A.J., Rempel, D.M., and Ames, B.N. (1996). Smoking and low antioxidant levels increase oxidative damage to sperm DNA. *Mutat. Res.* 351, 199–203.

Freedman, D.A., Gold, L.S., and Lin, T.H. (1996). Concordance between rats and mice in bioassays for carcinogenesis. *Regul. Toxicol. Pharmacol.* 23, 225–232. http://www.idealibrary.com/links/doi/10.1006/rtph.1996.0046/pdf.

Freedman, D.A., Gold, L.S., and Slone, T.H. (1993). How tautological are inter-species correlations of carcinogenic potency? *Risk Anal.* 13, 265–272.

Freedman, D.A., and Zeisel, H. (1988). From mouse to man: The quantitative assessment of cancer risks. *Stat. Sci.* 3, 3–56.

Freidman, G.D., and Habel, L.A. (1999). Barbiturates and lung cancer: A re-evaluation. *Int. J. Cancer* 28, 375–379.

Gaido, K., Dohme, L., Wang, F., Chen, I., Blankvoort, B., Ramamoorthy, K., and Safe, S. (1998). Comparative estrogenic activity of wine extracts and organochlorine pesticide residues in food. *Environ. Health Perspect.* 106 (Suppl. 6), 1347–1351.

Galanis, D.J., Kolonel, L.N., Lee, J., and Nomura, A. (1998). Intakes of selected foods and beverages and the incidence of gastric cancer among the Japanese residents of Hawaii: A prospective study. *Int. J. Epidemiol.* 27, 173–180.

Gammon, M.D., Wolff, M.S., Neugut, A.I., Eng, S.M., Teitelbaum, S.L., Britton, J.A., Terry, M.B., Levin, B., Stellman, S.D., Kabat, G.C., Hatch, M., Senie, R., Berkowitz, G., Bradlow, H.L., Garbowski, G., Maffeo, C., Montalvan, P., Kemeny, M., Citron, M., Schnabel, F., Schuss, A., Hajdu, S., Vinceguerra, V., Niguidula, N., Ireland, K., and Santella, R.M. (2002). Environmental Toxins and Breast Cancer on Long Island. II. Organochlorine Compound Levels in Blood. *Cancer Epidemiol. Biomarkers Prev.* 11, 686–697.

Gartrell, M.J., Craun, J.C., Podrebarac, D.S., and Gunderson, E.L. (1986). Pesticides, selected elements, and other chemicals in adult total diet samples, October 1980–March 1982. *J. Assoc. Off. Anal. Chem.* 69, 146–161.

Gaylor, D.W., Chen, J.J., and Sheehan, D.M. (1993). Uncertainty in cancer risk estimates. *Risk Anal.* 13, 149–154.

Gaylor, D.W., and Gold, L.S. (1995). Quick estimate of the regulatory virtually safe dose based on the maximum tolerated dose for rodent bioassays. *Regul. Toxicol. Pharmacol.* 22, 57–63. doi:10.1006/rtph.1995.1069.

Gaylor, D.W., and Gold, L.S. (1998). Regulatory cancer risk assessment based an a quick estimate of a benchmark dose derived from the maximum tolerated dose. *Regul. Toxicol. Pharmacol.* 28, 222–225. doi: 10.1006/rtph.1998.1258.

Giovannucci, E., Ascherio, A., Rimm, E.B., Colditz, G.A., Stampfer, M.J., and Willett, W.C. (1995). Physical activity, obesity, and risk of colon cancer and adenoma in men. *Ann. Intern. Med.* 122, 327–334.

Giovannucci, E., Colditz, G.A., Stampfer, M.J., and Willett, W.C. (1996). Physical activity, obesity, and risk of colorectal adenoma in women (United States). *Cancer Causes Control* 7, 253–263.

Giovannucci, E., Rimm, E.B., Liu, Y., and Stampfer, M.J. (2002). A prospective study of tomato products, lycopene, and prostate cancer risk. *J. Natl. Cancer Inst.* 94, 391–398.

Giovannucci, E., Stampfer, M.J., Colditz, G.A., Hunter, D.J., Fuchs, C., Rosner, B.A., Speizer, F.E., and Willett, W.C. (1998). Multivitamin use, folate, and colon cancer in women in the Nurses' Health Study. *Ann. Intern. Med.* 129, 517–524.

Giovannucci, E., Stampfer, M.J., Colditz, G.A., Rimm, E.B., Trichopoulos, D., Rosner, B.A., Speizer, F.E., and Willett, W.C. (1993). Folate, methionine, and alcohol intake and risk of colorectal adenoma. *J. Natl. Cancer Inst.* 85, 875–884.

Glória, M.B.A., Barbour, J.F., and Scanlan, R.A. (1997). N-nitrosodimethylamine in Brazilian, US domestic, and US imported beers. *J. Agric. Food Chem.* 45, 814–816.

Gold, L.S., Backman, G.M., Hooper, N.K., and Peto, R. (1987a). Ranking the potential carcinogenic hazards to workers from exposures to chemicals that are tumorigenic in rodents. *Environ. Health Perspect.* 76, 211–219.

Gold, L.S., Wright, C., Bernstein, L., and de Veciana, M. (1987b). Reproducibility of results in "near-replicate" carcinogenesis bioassays. *J. Natl. Cancer Inst.* 78, 1149–1158.

Gold, L.S., Bernstein, L., Magaw, R., and Slone, T.H. (1989a). Interspecies extrapolation in carcinogenesis: Prediction between rats and mice. *Environ. Health Perspect.* 81, 211–219.

Gold, L.S., Slone, T.H., and Bernstein, L. (1989b). Summary of carcinogenic potency (TD_{50}) and positivity for 492 rodent carcinogens in the Carcinogenic Potency Database. *Environ. Health Perspect.* 79, 259–272.

Gold, L.S., Slone, T.H., Stern, B.R., Manley, N.B., and Ames, B.N. (1992). Rodent carcinogens: Setting priorities. *Science* 258, 261–265. http://potency.berkeley.edu/text/science.html.

Gold, L.S., Garfinkel, G.B., and Slone, T.H. (1994a). Setting priorities among possible carcinogenic hazards in the workplace. In *Chemical Risk Assessment and Occupational Health: Current Applications, Limitations, and Future Prospects* (C.M. Smith, D.C. Christiani and K.T. Kelsey, eds.), pp. 91–103. Auburn House, Westport, CT.

Gold, L.S., Slone, T.H., Manley, N.B., and Ames, B.N. (1994b). Heterocyclic amines formed by cooking food: Comparison of bioassay results with other chemicals in the Carcinogenic Potency Database. *Cancer Lett.* 83, 21–29.

Gold, L.S., and Zeiger, E., eds. (1997). *Handbook of Carcinogenic Potency and Genotoxicity Databases.* CRC Press, Boca Raton, FL. http://potency.berkeley.edu/crcbook.html.

Gold, L.S., Slone, T.H., and Ames, B.N. (1997a). Overview of Analyses of the Carcinogenic Potency Database. In *Handbook of Carcinogenic Potency and Genotoxicity Databases* (L.S. Gold and E. Zeiger, eds.), pp. 661–685. CRC Press, Boca Raton, FL.

Gold, L.S., Slone, T.H., and Ames, B.N. (1997b). Prioritization of possible carcinogenic hazards in food. In *Food Chemical Risk Analysis* (D.R. Tennant, ed.), pp. 267–295. Chapman and Hall, London. http://potency.berkeley.edu/text/maff.html.

Gold, L.S., Slone, T.H., Ames, B.N., Manley, N.B., Garfinkel, G.B., and Rohrbach, L. (1997c). Carcinogenic Potency Database. In *Handbook of Carcinogenic Potency and Genotoxicity Databases* (L. S. Gold and E. Zeiger, eds.), pp. 1–605. CRC Press, Boca Raton, FL. http://potency.berkeley.edu/database.html.

Gold, L.S., Stern, B.R., Slone, T.H., Brown, J.P., Manley, N.B., and Ames, B.N. (1997d). Pesticide residues in food: Investigation of disparities in cancer risk estimates. *Cancer Lett.* 117, 195–207. http://potency.berkeley.edu/text/pesticide.html.

Gold, L.S., Slone, T.H., and Ames, B.N. (1998). What do animal cancer tests tell us about human cancer risk? Overview of analyses of the Carcinogenic Potency Database. *Drug Metab. Rev.* 30, 359–404. http://potency.berkeley.edu/text/drugmetrev.html.

Gold, L.S., Manley, N.B., Slone, T.H., and Rohrbach, L. (1999). Supplement to the Carcinogenic Potency Database (CPDB): Results of animal bioassays published in the general literature in 1993 to 1994 and by the National Toxicology Program in 1995 to 1996. *En-*

viron. *Health Perspect.* 107 (Suppl. 4), 527–600. http://ehpnet1.niehs.nih.gov/docs/1999/suppl-4/toc.html.

Gold, L.S., Manley, N.B., Slone, T.H., and Ward, J.M. (2001a). Compendium of chemical carcinogens by target organ: Results of chronic bioassays in rats, mice, hamsters, dogs and monkeys. *Toxicol. Pathol.* 29, 639–652.

Gold, L.S., Slone, T.H., Ames, B.N., and Manley, N.B. (2001b). Pesticide residues in food and cancer risk: A critical analysis. In *Handbook of Pesticide Toxicology* (R.I. Krieger, ed.), Vol. 1, pp. 799–843. Academic Press, New York.

Goodman, D.G., and Sauer, R.M. (1992). Hepatotoxicity and carcinogenicity in female Sprague-Dawley rats treated with 2,3,7,8-tetrachlorodibenzo-p-dioxin (TCDD): A pathology working group reevaluation. *Regul. Toxicol. Pharmacol.* 15, 245–252.

Goodman, J.I. (1994). A rational approach to risk assessment requires the use of biological information: An Analysis of the National Toxicology Program (NTP), final report of the advisory review by the NTP Board of Scientific Counselors. *Regul. Toxicol. Pharmacol.* 19, 51–59.

Gough, M. (1990). How much cancer can EPA regulate away? *Risk Anal.* 10, 1–6.

Graham, J.D., and Wiener, J.B., eds. (1995). *Risk versus Risk: Tradeoffs in Protecting Health and the Environment.* Harvard University Press, Cambridge, MA.

Gray-Donald, K., Jacobs-Starkey, L., and Johnson-Down, L. (2000). Food habits of Canadians: Reduction in fat intake over a generation. *Can. J. Public Health* 91, 381–385.

Gribble, G.W. (1996). The diversity of natural organochlorines in living organisms. *Pure Appl. Chem.* 68, 1699–1712.

Grodstein, F., Stampfer, M.J., Colditz, G.A., Willett, W.C., Manson, J.E., Joffe, M., Rosner, B., Fuchs, C., Hankinson, S.E., Hunter, D.J., Hennekens, C.H., and Speizer, F.E. (1997). Postmenopausal hormone therapy and mortality. *N. Engl. J. Med.* 336, 1769–1775.

Groopman, J.D., Zhu, J.Q., Donahue, P.R., Pikul, A., Zhang, L.S., Chen, J.S., and Wogan, G.N. (1992). Molecular dosimetry of urinary aflatoxin-DNA adducts in people living in Guangxi Autonomous Region, People's Republic of China. *Cancer Res.* 52, 45–52.

Gruenwald, J., Brendler, T., and Jaenicke, C., eds. (1998). *PDR for Herbal Medicines.* Medical Economics Company, Montvale, NJ.

Guallar, E., and Goodman, S.N. (2001). Statins and cancer: A case of meta-uncertainty. *Am. J. Med.* 110, 738–740.

Gunawardhana, L., Mobley, S.A., and Sipes, I.G. (1993). Modulation of 1,2-dichlorobenzene hepatotoxicity in the Fischer-344 rat by a scavenger of superoxide anions and an inhibitor of Kupffer cells. *Toxicol. Appl. Pharmacol.* 119, 205–213.

Gunderson, E.L. (1995). Dietary intakes of pesticides, selected elements, and other chemicals: FDA Total Diet Study, June 1984–April 1986. *J. Assoc. Off. Anal. Chem.* 78, 910–921.

Gyllenborg, J., Skakkebaek, N.E., Nielsen, N.C., Keiding, N., and Giwercman, A. (1999). Secular and seasonal changes in semen quality among young Danish men: a statistical analysis of semen samples from 1,927 donor candidates during 1977–1995. *Int. J. Androl.* 22, 28–36.

Hagen, T.M., Liu, J., Lykkesfeldt, J., Wehr, C.M., Ingersoll, R.T., Vinarsky, V., Bartholomew, J.C., and Ames, B.N. (2002). Feeding acetyl-L-carnitine and lipoic acid to old rats significantly improves metabolic function while decreasing oxidative stress. *Proc. Natl. Acad. Sci. USA* 99, 1870–1875.

Hagen, T.M., Yowe, D.L., Bartholomew, J.C., Wehr, C.M., Do, K.L., Park, J.-Y., and Ames, B.N. (1997). Mitochondrial decay in hepatocytes from old rats: Membrane potential declines, heterogeneity and oxidants increase. *Proc. Natl. Acad. Sci. USA* 94, 3064–3069.

Hahn, R.W., ed. (1996). *Risks, Costs, and Lives Saved: Getting Better Results from Regulation.* Oxford University Press, New York.

Hahn, R.W., and Stavins, R.N. (2001). *National Environmental Policy During the Clinton Years 1992–2000.* Harvard University, Cambridge, MA.

Hall, R.L., Henry, S.H., Scheuplein, R.J., Dull, B.J., and Rulis, A.M. (1989). Comparison of the carcinogenic risks of naturally occurring and adventitious substances in food. In *Food Toxicology: A Perspective on the Relative Risks* (S. L. Taylor and R. A. Scanlan, eds.), pp. 205–224. Marcel Dekker, New York.

Hard, G.C., and Whysner, J. (1994). Risk assessment of d-limonene: An example of male rat-specific renal tumorigens. *Crit. Rev. Toxicol.* 24, 231–254.

Hart, R., Neumann, D., and Robertson, R. (1995a). *Dietary Restriction: Implications for the Design and Interpretation of Toxicity and Carcinogenicity Studies.* ILSI Press, Washington, DC.

Hart, R.W., Keenan, K., Turturro, A., Abdo, K.M., Leakey, J., and Lyn-Cook, B. (1995b). Caloric restriction and toxicity. *Fundam. Appl. Toxicol.* 25, 184–195.

Havel, R.J., and Kane, J.P. (1982). Therapy of hyperlipidemic states. *Ann. Rev. Med.* 33, 417.

Hayashi, F., Tamura, H., Yamada, J., Kasai, H., and Suga, T. (1994). Characteristics of the hepatocarcinogenesis caused by dehydroepiandrosterone, a peroxisome proliferator, in male F-344 rats. *Carcinogenesis* 15, 2215–2219.

Health Canada (1995). *Drugs Directorate Policy on Herbals used as Non-medicinal Ingredients in Nonprescription*

Drugs in Human Use, Vol. 2001. Health Canada. http://www.hc-sc.gc.ca/hpb-dgps/therapeut/zfiles/english/policy/issued/herbnmi_e.html.

Health Canada (1998). *Mandatory Fortification of Flour and Pasta with Folic Acid. Schedule 1066.* Health Canada, Toronto, Canada.

Health Canada (2000). *Food and Drugs Act and Regulations, Vol. 2001.* Health Canada. http://www.hc-sc.gc.ca/food-aliment/english/publications/acts_and_regulations/food_and_drugs_acts/index.html.

Hecht, S.S., and Hoffmann, D. (1998). N-nitroso compounds and man: sources of exposure, endogenous formation and occurrence in body fluids. *Eur. J. Cancer Prev.* 7, 165–166.

Heddle, J.A. (1998). The role of proliferation in the origin of mutations in mammalian cells. *Drug Metab. Rev.* 30, 327–338.

Heinrich, L., and Baltes, W. (1987). Über die Bestimmung von Phenolen im Kaffeegetränk. *Z. Lebensm. Unters. Forsch.* 185, 362–365.

Helbock, H.J., Beckman, K.B., Shigenaga, M.K., Walter, P.B., Woodall, A.A., Yeo, H.C., and Ames, B.N. (1998). DNA oxidation matters: The HPLC–electrochemical detection assay of 8-oxo-deoxyguanosine and 8-oxo-guanine. *Proc. Natl. Acad. Sci. USA* 95, 288–293.

Henderson, B.E., and Feigelson, H.S. (2000). Hormonal carcinogenesis. *Carcinogenesis* 21, 427–33.

Henderson, B.E., Ross, R.K., and Pike, M.C. (1991). Towards the primary prevention of cancer. *Science* 254, 1131–1138.

Herbert, V., and Filer, L.J., Jr. (1996). Vitamin B–12. In *Present Knowledge in Nutrition* (E. E. Ziegler, ed.), pp. 191–205. ILSI Press, Washington, DC.

Herrmann, K. (1978). Review on nonessential constituents of vegetables. III. Carrots, celery, parsnips, beets, spinach, lettuce, endives, chicory, rhubarb, and artichokes. *Z. Lebensm. Unters. Forsch.* 167, 262–273.

Hill, L.L., Ouhtit, A., Loughlin, S.M., Kripke, M.L., Ananthaswamy, H.N., and Owen–Schaub, L.B. (1999). Fas ligand: A sensor for DNA damage critical in skin cancer etiology. *Science* 285, 898–900.

Hill, M.J., Giacosa, A., and Caygill, C.P.J., eds. (1994). *Epidemiology of Diet and Cancer.* Ellis Horwood, New York.

Hirono, I., Mori, H., and Haga, M. (1978). Carcinogenic activity of *Symphytum officinale*. *J. Natl. Cancer Inst.* 61, 865–868.

Huang, Z., Hankinson, S.E., Colditz, G.A., Stampfer, M.J., Hunter, D.J., Manson, J.E., Hennekens, C.H., Rosner, B., Speizer, F.E., and Willett, W.C. (1997). Dual effects of weight and weight gain on breast cancer risk. *JAMA* 278, 1407–1411.

Hunter, D.J., Spiegelman, D., Adami, H.O., Beeson, L., van den Brandt, P.A., Folsom, A.R., Fraser, G.E., Goldbohm, R.A., Graham, S., Howe, G.R., Kushi, L.H., Marshall, J.R., McDermott, A., Miller, A.B., Speizer, F.E., Wolk, A., Yaun, S.-S., and Willett, W.C. (1996). Cohort studies of fat intake and the risk of breast cancer—a pooled analysis. *N. Engl. J. Med.* 334, 356–361.

Hunter, D.J., Spiegelman, D., and Willett, W. (1998). Dietary fat and breast cancer. *J. Natl. Cancer Inst.* 90, 1303–1306.

Hunter, D.J., and Willett, W.C. (1993). Diet, body size, and breast cancer. *Epidemiol. Rev.* 15, 110–132.

Huxtable, R. (1995). Pyrrolizidine alkaloids: Fascinating plant poisons. *Newsletter, Center for Toxicology, Southwest Environmental Health Sciences Center* Fall, 1–3.

Ince, N., and Wands, J.R. (1999). The increasing incidence of hepatocellular carcinoma. *N. Engl. J. Med.* 340, 798–799.

Innes, J.R.M., Ulland, B.M., Valerio, M.G., Petrucelli, L., Fishbein, L., Hart, E.R., Pallota, A.J., Bates, R.R., Falk, H.L., Gart, J.J., Klein, M., Mitchell, I., and Peters, J. (1969).

Bioassay of pesticides and industrial chemicals for tumorigenicity in mice: A preliminary note. *J. Natl. Cancer Inst.* 42, 1101–1114.

International Agency for Research on Cancer (1971–2001). *IARC Monographs on the Evaluation of Carcinogenic Risk of Chemicals to Humans.* IARC, Lyon, France.

International Agency for Research on Cancer (1971–2002). *IARC Monographs on the Evaluation of Carcinogenic Risk of Chemicals to Humans.* IARC, Lyon, France.

International Agency for Research on Cancer (1986). *Tobacco Smoking.* IARC, Lyon, France.

International Agency for Research on Cancer (1988). *Alcohol Drinking.* IARC, Lyon, France.

International Agency for Research on Cancer (1991). *Coffee, Tea, Mate, Methylxanthines and Methylglyoxal.* IARC, Lyon, France.

International Agency for Research on Cancer (1993). *Some Naturally Occurring Substances: Food Items, Constituents, and Heterocyclic Aromatic Amines and Mycotoxins.* IARC, Lyon, France.

International Agency for Research on Cancer (1996). *Some Pharmaceutical Drugs.* IARC, Lyon, France.

International Agency for Research on Cancer (1997). *Polychlorinated Dibenzo–para–dioxins and Polychlorinated Dibenzofurans.* IARC, Lyon, France.

International Agency for Research on Cancer (1999a). *Re-Evaluation of Some Organic Chemicals, Hydrazine and Hydrogen Peroxide.* IARC, Lyon, France.

International Agency for Research on Cancer (1999b). *Some Chemicals That Cause Tumours of the Kidney or Urinary Bladder in Rodents and Some Other Substances.* IARC, Lyon, France.

International Agency for Research on Cancer (2002, in press). *Tobacco Smoke and Involuntary Smoking.* IARC, Lyon, France.

International Life Sciences Institute (February 1996). Occurrence and significance of ochratoxin A in food. ILSI Europe Workshop, 10–12 January 1996, Aix–en–Provence, France. *ILSI Europe Newsletter,* 3.

Ivie, G.W., Holt, D.L., and Ivey, M. (1981). Natural toxicants in human foods: Psoralens in raw and cooked parsnip root. *Science* 213, 909–910.

Jacobson, E.L. (1993). Niacin deficiency and cancer in women. *J. Am. Coll. Nutr.* 12, 412–416.

Jacques, P.F., Selhub, J., Bostom, A.G., Wilson, P.W., and Rosenberg, I.H. (1999). The effect of folic acid fortification on plasma folate and total homocysteine concentrations. *N. Engl. J. Med.* 340, 1449–1454.

Jansen, M.C.J.F., Bueno-de-Mesquita, H.B., Räsänen, L., Fidanza, F., Nissinen, A.M., Menotti, A., Kok, F.J., and Kromhout, D. (2001). Cohort analysis of fruit and vegetable consumption and lung cancer mortality in European men. *Int. J. Cancer* 92, 913–918.

Japanese Environmental Agency (1999). *Report on the Tolerable Daily Intake (TDI) of Dioxin and Related Compounds.* Ministry of Health and Welfare, Tokyo.

Ji, B.-T., Shu, X.-O., Linet, M.S., Zheng, W., Wacholder, S., Gao, Y.-T., Ying, D.-M., and Jin, F. (1997). Paternal cigarette smoking and the risk of childhood cancer among offspring of nonsmoking mothers. *J. Natl. Cancer Inst.* 89, 238–244.

Jukes, T.H. (1974). DDT. *JAMA* 229, 571–573.

Kasum, C.M., Jacobs, D.R., Jr., Nicodemus, K., and Folsom, A.R. (2002). Dietary risk factors for upper aerodigestive tract cancers. *Int. J. Cancer* 99, 267–272.

Keating, G.A., and Bogen, K.T. (2001). Methods for estimating heterocyclic amine concentrations in cooked meats in the US diet. *Food Chem. Toxicol.* 39, 29–43.

Keeney, R.L. (1990). Mortality risks induced by economic expenditures. *Risk Anal.* 10, 147–159.

Kelloff, G.J., Boone, C.W., Crowell, J.A., Steele, V.E., Lubet, R.A., Doody, L.A., Malone, W.F., Hawk, E.T., and Sigman, C.C. (1996a). New agents for cancer chemoprevention. *J. Cell Biochem. Suppl.* 26, 1–28.

Kelloff, G.J., Crowell, J.A., Hawk, E.T., Steele, V.E., Lubet, R.A., Boone, C.W., Covey, J.M., Doody, L.A., Omenn, G.S., Greenwald, P., Hong, W.K., Parkinson, D.R., Bagheri, D., Baxter, G.T., Blunden, M., Doeltz, M.K., Eisenhauer, K.M., Johnson, K., Knapp, G.G., Longfellow, G., Malone, W.F., Nayfield, S.G., Seifried, H.E., Swall, L.M., and Sigman, C.C. (1996b). Strategy and planning for chemopreventive drug development: Clinical development plans II. *J. Cell Biochem. Suppl.* 26, 54–71.

Kelsey, J.L., and Bernstein, L. (1996). Epidemiology and prevention of breast cancer. *Annu. Rev. Public Health* 17, 47–67.

Key, T., and Reeves, G. (1994). Organochlorines in the environment and breast cancer. *Br. Med. J.* 308, 1520–1521.

Knize, M.G., Dolbeare, F.A., Carroll, K.L., Moore II, D.H., and Felton, J.S. (1994). Effect of cooking time and temperature on the heterocyclic amine content of fried beef patties. *Food Chem. Toxicol.* 32, 595–603.

Kolata, G. (1996). Measuring men up, sperm by sperm. In *New York Times*, Vol. 145, pp. E4(N), E4(L).

Krebs-Smith, S.M., Cook, A., Subar, A.F., Cleveland, L., and Friday, J. (1995). US adults' fruit and vegetable intakes, 1989 to 1991: A revised baseline for the Healthy People 2000 objective. *Am. J. Public Health* 85, 1623–1629.

Krebs-Smith, S.M., Cook, A., Subar, A.F., Cleveland, L., Friday, J., and Kahle, L.L. (1996). Fruit and vegetable intakes of children and adolescents in the United States. *Arch. Pediatr. Adolesc. Med.* 150, 81–86.

Krul, C., Humblot, C., Philippe, C., Vermeulen, M., van Nuenen, M., Havenaar, R., and Rabot, S. (2002). Metabolism of sinigrin (2-propenyl glucosinolate) by the human colonic microflora in a dynamic *in vitro* large-intestinal model. *Carcinogenesis* 23, 1009–1016.

Kuiper-Goodman, T., and Scott, P.M. (1989). Risk assessment of the mycotoxin ochratoxin A. *Biomed. Environ. Sci.* 2, 179–248.

Laden, F., Hankinson, S.E., Wolff, M.S., Colditz, G.A., Willett, W.C., Speizer, F.E., and Hunter, D.J. (2001). Plasma organochlorine levels and the risk of breast cancer: An extended follow–up in the Nurses' Health Study. *Int. J. Cancer* 91, 568–574.

Laskin, D.L., and Pendino, K.J. (1995). Macrophages and inflammatory mediators in tissue injury. *Annu. Rev. Pharmacol. Toxicol.* 35, 655–677.

Laskin, D.L., Robertson, F.M., Pilaro, A.M., and Laskin, J.D. (1988). Activation of liver macrophages following phenobarbital treatment of rats. *Hepatology* 8, 1051–1055.

Lau, V.K., and Lindsay, R.C. (1972). Quantification of monocarbonyl compounds in staling beer. *Master Brew. Assoc. Am. Tech. Q.* 9, xvii–xviii.

Lijinsky, W. (1999). *N*-Nitroso compounds in the diet. *Mutat. Res.* 443, 129–138.

Lin, T.H., Gold, L.S., and Freedman, D.A. (1995). Carcinogenicity tests and interspecies concordance. *Stat. Sci.* 10, 337–353.

Linet, M.S., Ries, L.A., Smith, M.A., Tarone, R.E., and Devesa, S.S. (1999). Cancer surveillance series: Recent trends in childhood cancer incidence and mortality in the United States. *J. Natl. Cancer Inst.* 91, 1051–1058.

Liu, J., Head, E., Gharib, A.M., Yuan, W., Ingersoll, R.T., Hagen, T.M., Cotman, C.W., and Ames, B.N. (2002a). Memory loss in old rats is associated with brain mitochondrial decay and RNA/DNA oxidation: Partial reversal by feeding acetyl-L-carnitine and/or R-α-lipoic acid. *Proc. Natl. Acad. Sci. USA* 99, 2356–2361.

Liu, J., Killilea, D.W., and Ames, B.N. (2002b). Age-associated mitochondrial oxidative decay: Improvement of carnitine acetyltransferase substrate-binding affinity and activity in brain by feeding old rats acetyl-L-carnitine and/or R-α-lipoic acid. *Proc. Natl. Acad. Sci. USA* 99, 1876–1881.

Lok, E., Scott, F.W., Mongeau, R., Nera, E.A., Malcolm, S., and Clayson, D.B. (1990). Calorie restriction and cellular proliferation in various tissues of the female Swiss Webster mouse. *Cancer Lett.* 51, 67–73.

Lucas, C.D., Putanm, J.D., and Hallagan, J.B. (1999). *1995 Poundage and Technical Effects Update Survey.* Flavor and Extract Manufacturer's Association of the United States, Washington, DC.

Luckey, T.D. (1999). Nurture with ionizing radiation: A provocative hypothesis. *Nutr. Cancer* 34, 1–11.

Lykkesfeldt, J., Christen, S., Walloock, L.M., Chang, H.H., Jacob, R.A., and Ames, B.N. (2000). Ascorbate is depleted by smoking and repleted by moderate supplementation: A study in male smokers and nonsmokers with matched dietary antioxidant intakes. *Am. J. Clin. Nutr.* 71, 530–536.

Makomaski Illing, E.M., and Kaiserman, M.J. (1999). Mortality attributable to tobacco use in Canada and its regions, 1994 and 1996. *Chronic Dis. Can.* 20, 111–117.

Manuel, D.G., and Hockin, J. (2000). Recent trends in provincial life expectancy. *Can. J. Public Health* 91, 118–119.

Marsh, G.M., Lucas, L.J., Youk, A.O., and Schall, L.C. (1999). Mortality patterns among workers exposed to acrylamide: 1994 follow up. *Occup. Environ. Med.* 56, 181–190.

Martinez, M.E., Giovannucci, E., Spiegelman, D., Hunter, D.J., Willett, W.C., and Colditz, G.A. (1997). Leisure-time physical activity, body size, and colon cancer in women. Nurses' Health Study Research Group. *J. Natl. Cancer Inst.* 89, 948–955.

Mason, J.B. (1994). Folate and colonic carcinogenesis: Searching for a mechanistic understanding. *J. Nutr. Biochem.* 5, 170–175.

Matanoski, G., Francis, M., Correa-Villaseñor, A., Elliot, E., Santos-Brugoa, C., and Schwartz, L. (1993). Cancer epidemiology among styrene–butadiene rubber workers. *IARC Sci. Pub.* 127, 363–374.

Matsumoto, K., Ito, M., Yagyu, S., Ogino, H., and Hirono, I. (1991). Carcinogenicity examination of *Agaricus bisporus*, edible mushroom, in rats. *Cancer Lett.* 58, 87–90.

McCann, J., Horn, L., Girman, J., and Nero, A.V. (1987). Potential risks from exposure to organic carcinogens in indoor air. In *Short-Term Bioassays in the Analysis of Complex Environmental Mixtures* (S.S. Sandhu, D.M. deMarini, M.J. Mass, M.M. Moore and J.L. Mumford, eds.), pp. 325–354. Plenum, New York.

McClain, R.M. (1990). Mouse liver tumors and microsomal enzyme–inducing drugs: experimental and clinical perspectives with phenobarbital. *Prog. Clin. Biol. Res.* 331, 345–365.

McClain, R.M. (1994). Mechanistic considerations in the regulation and classification of chemical carcinogens. In *Nutritional Toxicology* (F.N. Kotsonis, M. Mackey and J.J. Hjelle, eds.), pp. 273–304. Raven Press, New York.

McCormick, D.L., Rao, K.V.N., Johnson, W.D., Bowman-Gram, T.A., Steele, V.E., Lubet, R.A., and Kelloff, G.J. (1996). Exceptional chemopreventive activity of low-dose dehydroepiandrosterone in the rat mammary gland. *Cancer Res.* 56, 1724–1726.

McCullough, M.L., Robertson, A.S., Jacobs, E.J., Chao, A., Calle, E.E., and Thun, M.J. (2001). A prospective study of diet and stomach cancer mortality in United States men and women. *Cancer Epidemiol. Biomarkers Prev.* 10, 1201–1205.

McKone, T.E. (1987). Human exposure to volatile organic compounds in household tap water: The indoor inhalation pathway. *Environ. Sci. Technol.* 21, 1194–1201.

McKone, T.E. (1993). Linking a PBPK model for chloroform with measured breath concentrations in showers: Implications for dermal exposure models. *J. Expo. Anal. Environ. Epidemiol.* 3, 339–365.

McLean, A.E.M., Driver, H.E., Lowe, D., and Sutherland, I. (1986). Thresholds for tumour promotion by phenobarbital after nitrosamine exposure in rat and man (Abstract). *Toxicol. Letters* 31 (Suppl.), 200.

Mengs, U. (1982). The carcinogenic action of aristolochic acid in rats. *Arch. Toxicol.* 51, 107–119.

Mengs, U. (1988). Tumour induction in mice following exposure to aristolochic acid. *Arch. Toxicol.* 61, 504–505.

Michels, K.B., Giovannucci, E., Joshipura, K.J., Rosner, B.A., Stampfer, M.J., Fuchs, C.S., Colditz, G.A., Speizer, F.E., and Willett, W.C. (2000). Prospective study of fruit and vegetable consumption and incidence of colon and rectal cancers. *J. Natl. Cancer Inst.* 92, 1740–1752.

Ministry of Environment and Energy (1997). *Green Facts: Environment and Energy Topics at a Glance. Dioxins and Furans.* Ministry of Environment and Energy, Toronto, Ontario. http://www.ene.gov.on.ca/cons/681e01.pdf.

Mosel, H.D., and Herrmann, K. (1974). The phenolics of fruits. III. The contents of catechins and hydroxycinnamic acids in pome and stone fruits. *Z. Lebensm. Unters. Forsch.* 154, 6–11.

Munday, R., and Munday, C.M. (1999). Low doses of diallyl disulfide, a compound derived from garlic, increase tissue activities of quinone reductase and glutathione transferase in the gastrointestinal tract of the rat. *Nutr. Cancer* 34, 42–48.

National Cancer Institute of Canada (2000). *Canadian Cancer Statistics 2000.* NCIC, Toronto, Canada.

National Cancer Institute of Canada (2001). *Canadian Cancer Statistics 2001.* NCIC, Toronto, Canada.

National Research Council (1979). *The 1977 Survey of Industry on the Use of Food Additives.* National Academy Press, Washington, DC.

National Research Council (1987). *Regulating Pesticides in Food: The Delaney Paradox.* National Academy Press, Washington, DC.

National Research Council (1996). *Carcinogens and Anticarcinogens in the Human Diet: A Comparison of Naturally Occurring and Synthetic Substances.* National Academy Press, Washington, DC.

National Research Council (1999). *Hormonally Active Agents in the Environment.* National Academy Press, Washington, DC.

Nephew, T.M., Williams, G.D., Stinson, F.S., Nguyen, K., and Dufour, M.C. (2000). *Surveillance Report #55: Apparent per Capita Alcohol Consumption: National, State and Regional Trends, 1977–1998.* National Institute on Alcohol Abuse and Alcoholism, Rockville, MD.

Neurath, G.B., Dünger, M., Pein, F.G., Ambrosius, D., and Schreiber, O. (1977). Primary and secondary amines in the human environment. *Food Cosmet. Toxicol.* 15, 275–282.

Newbold, R.R., Banks, E.P., Bullock, B., and Jefferson, W.N. (2001). Uterine adenocarcinoma in mice treated neonatally with genistein. *Cancer Res.* 61, 4325–4328.

Nijssen, L.M., Visscher, C.A., Maarse, H., Willemsens, L.C., and Boelens, M.H., eds. (1996). *Volatile Compounds in Foods. Qualitative and Quantitative Data.* TNO–CIVO Food Analysis Institute, Zeist, The Netherlands.

Nortier, J.L., Muniz Martinez, M.-C., Schmeiser, H.H., Arlt, V.M., Bieler, C.A., Petein, M., Depierreux, M.F., De Pauw, L., Abramowicz, D., Vereerstraeten, P., and Vanherweghem, J.-L. (2000). Urothelial carcinoma associated with the use of a Chinese herb (*Aristolochia fangchi*). *N. Engl. J. Med.* 342, 1686–1692.

Oelkers, W. (1999). Dehydroepiandrosterone for adrenal insufficiency. *N. Engl. J. Med.* 341, 1073–1074.

Ogawa, K., Tsuda, H., Shirai, T., Ogiso, T., Wakabayashi, K., Dalgard, D.W., Thorgeirsson, U.P., Thorgeirsson, S.S., Adamson, R.H., and Sugimura, T. (1999). Lack of carcinogenicity of 2-amino-3,8-dimethylimidazo[4,5-*f*]quinoxaline (MeIQx) in cynomolgus monkeys. *Jpn. J. Cancer Res.* 90, 622–628.

Omenn, G.S., Stuebbe, S., and Lave, L.B. (1995). Predictions of rodent carcinogenicity testing results: Interpretation in light of the Lave-Omenn value-of-information model. *Mol. Carcinog.* 14, 37–45.

Osler, M., Tjonneland, A., Suntum, M., Thomsen, B.L., Stripp, C., Gronbaek, M., and Overvad, K. (2002). Does the association between smoking status and selected healthy foods depend on gender? A population-based study of 54,417 middle–aged Danes. *Eur. J. Clin. Nutr.* 56, 57–63.

Ott, M.G., Scharnweber, H.C., and Langner, R.R. (1980). Mortality experience of 161 employees exposed to ethylene dibromide in two production units. *Br. J. Ind. Med.* 37, 163–168.

Ozasa, K., Watanabe, Y., Ito, Y., Suzuki, K., Tamakoshi, A., Seki, N., Nishino, Y., Kondo, T., Wakai, K., Ando, M., and Ohno, Y. (2001). Dietary habits and risk of lung cancer death in a large–scale cohort study (JACC Study) in Japan by sex and smoking habit. *Jpn. J. Cancer Res.* 92, 1259–1269.

Page, N.P., and Arthur, J.L. (1978). *Special Occupational Hazard Review of Trichloroethylene*. National Institute for Occupational Safety and Health, Rockville, MD.

Patterson, R.E., Kristal, A.R., and Neuhouser, M.L. (2001). Vitamin supplements and cancer risk: Epidemiologic research and recommendations. In *Primary and Secondary Preventive Nutrition* (A. Bendich and R. J. Deckelbau, eds.), pp. 21–43. Humana Press, Totowa, NJ.

Paustenbach, D.J. (2002, in press). Dioxin risks in perspective: past, present and future. *Regul. Toxicol. Pharmacol.* 36.

Peto, R., Boreham, J., Clarke, M., Davies, C., and Beral, V. (2000). UK and USA breast cancer deaths down 25% in year 2000 at ages 20–69 years. *Lancet* 355, 1822.

Pfeffer, M.A., Keech, A., Sacks, F.M., Cobbe, S.M., Tonkin, A., Byington, R.P., Davis, B.R., Friedman, C.P., and Braunwald, E. (2002). Safety and tolerability of pravastatin in long-term clinical trials: prospective Pravastatin Pooling (PPP) Project. *Circulation* 105, 2341–2346.

Pisani, P., Parkin, D.M., Muñoz, N., and Ferlay, J. (1997). Cancer and infection: Estimates of the attributable fraction in 1990. *Cancer Epidemiol. Biomarkers Prev.* 6, 387–400.

Platz, E.A., Willett, W.C., Colditz, G.A., Rimm, E.B., Spiegelman, D., and Giovannucci, E. (2000). Proportion of colon cancer risk that might be preventable in a cohort of middle-aged US men. *Cancer Causes Control* 11, 579–588.

Podrebarac, D.S. (1984). Pesticide, metal, and other chemical residues in adult total diet samples. (XIV). October 1977–September 1978. *J. Assoc. Off. Anal. Chem.* 67, 176–185.

Pons, W.A., Jr. (1979). High pressure liquid chromatographic determination of aflatoxins in corn. *J. Assoc. Off. Anal. Chem.* 62, 586–594.

Poole, S.K., and Poole, C.F. (1994). Thin-layer chromatographic method for the determination of the principal polar aromatic flavour compounds of the cinnamons of commerce. *Analyst* 119, 113–120.

Prakash, A.S., Pereira, T.N., Reilly, P.E.B., and Seawright, A.A. (1999). Pyrrolizidine alkaloids in human diet. *Mutat. Res.* 443, 53–57.

Preussmann, R., and Eisenbrand, G. (1984). *N*-nitroso carcinogens in the environment. In *Chemical Carcino-*

genesis (C. E. Searle, ed.), Vol. 2, pp. 829–868. American Chemical Society (ACS), Washington DC.

Qian, G.-S., Ross, R.K., Yu, M.C., Yuan, J.-M., Henderson, B.E., Wogan, G.N., and Groopman, J.D. (1994). A follow-up study of urinary markers of aflatoxin exposure and liver cancer risk in Shanghai, People's Republic of China. *Cancer Epidemiol. Biomarkers Prev.* 3, 3–10.

Rahn, W., and König, W.A. (1978). GC/MS investigations of the constituents in a diethyl ether extract of an acidified roast coffee infusion. *J. High Resolut. Chromatogr. Chromatogr. Commun.* 1002, 69–71.

Ramsey, J.C., Park, C.N., Ott, M.G., and Gehring, P.J. (1978). Carcinogenic risk assessment: Ethylene dibromide. *Toxicol. Appl. Pharmacol.* 47, 411–414.

Rao, M.S., Subbarao, V., Yeldandi, A.V., and Reddy, J.K. (1992). Inhibition of spontaneous testicular Leydig cell tumor development in F-344 rats by dehydroepiandrosterone. *Cancer Lett.* 65.

Rao, M.S., Subbarao, V., Yeldandi, A.V., and Reddy, J.K. (1992). Hepatocarcinogenicity of dehydroepiandrosterone in the rat. *Cancer Res.* 52, 2977–2979.

Reddy, J.K., and Lalwani, N.D. (1983). Carcinogenesis by hepatic peroxisome proliferators: Evaluation of the risk of hypolipidemic drugs and industrial plasticizers to humans. *CRC Crit. Rev. Toxicol.* 12, 1–58.

Reid, D.P. (1993). *Chinese Herbal Medicine.* Shambhala, Boston.

Reinli, K., and Block, G. (1996). Phytoestrogen content of foods—a compendium of literature values. *Nutr. Cancer* 26, 123–148.

Rice, J.M., Baan, R.A., Blettner, M., Genevois-Charmeau, C., Grosse, Y., McGregor, D.B., Partensky, C., and Wilbourn, J.D. (1999). Rodent tumors of urinary bladder, renal cortex, and thyroid gland in IARC Monographs evaluations of carcinogenic risk to humans. *Toxicol. Sci.* 49, 166–171.

Rice–Evans, C.A., Sampson, J., Bramley, P.M., and Holloway, D.E. (1997). Why do we expect carotenoids to be antioxidants in vivo? *Free Rad. Res.* 26, 381–398.

Ries, L.A.G., Eisner, M.P., Kosary, C.L., Hankey, B.F., Miller, B.A., Clegg, L., and Edwards, B.K., eds. (2000). *SEER Cancer Statistics Review, 1973–1997.* National Cancer Institute, Bethesda, MD.

Roberts, R.A., and Kimber, I. (1999). Cytokines in nongenotoxic hepatocarcinogenesis. *Carcinogenesis* 20, 1397–1401.

Robisch, G., Schimmer, O., and Gogglemann, W. (1982). Aristolochic acid is a direct mutagen in *Salmonella typhimurium*. *Mutat. Res.* 105, 201–204.

Rockhill, B., Willett, W.C., Hunter, D.J., Manson, J.E., Hankinson, S.E., and Colditz, G.A. (1999). A prospective study of recreational physical activity and breast cancer risk. *Arch. Intern. Med.* 159, 2290–2296.

Rosenkranz, H.S., and Klopman, G. (1990). The structural basis of carcinogenic and mutagenic potentials of phytoalexins. *Mutat. Res.* 245, 51–54.

Safe, S., Wang, F., Porter, W., Duan, R., and McDougal, A. (1998). Ah receptor agonists as endocrine disruptors: Antiestrogenic activity and mechanisms. *Toxicol. Lett.* 102–103, 343–347.

Safe, S.H. (1995). Environmental and dietary estrogens and human health: Is there a problem? *Environ. Health Perspect.* 103, 346–351.

Safe, S.H. (1997). Is there an association between exposure to environmental estrogens and breast cancer? *Environ. Health Perspect.* 105 (Suppl. 3), 675–578.

Safe, S.H. (2000). Endocrine disruptors and human health—Is there a problem? An update. *Environ. Health Perspect.* 108, 487–493.

Saidi, J.A., Chang, D.T., Goluboff, E.T., Bagiella, E., Olsen, G., and Fisch, H. (1999). Declining sperm counts in the United States? A critical review. *J. Urol.* 161, 460–462.

Schecter, A., Cramer, P., Boggess, K., Stanley, J., Papke, O., Olson, J., Silver, A., and Schmitz, M. (2001). Intake of dioxins and related compounds from food in the U.S. population. *J. Toxicol. Environ. Health A* 63, 1–18.

Schmidtlein, H., and Herrmann, K. (1975a). Über die Phenolsäuren des Gemüses. II. Hydroxyzimtsäuren und Hydroxybenzoesäuren der Frucht- und Samengemüsearten. *Z. Lebensm. Unters.-Forsch.* 159, 213–218.

Schmidtlein, H., and Herrmann, K. (1975b). Über die Phenolsäuren des Gemüses. IV. Hydroxyzimtsäuren und Hydroxybenzösäuren weiterer Gemüsearten und der Kartoffeln. *Z. Lebensm. Unters. Forsch.* 159, 255–263.

Schreier, P., Drawert, F., and Heindze, I. (1979). Über die quantitative Zusammensetzung natürlicher und technologish veränderter pflanzlicher Aromen. *Chem. Mikrobiol. Technol. Lebensm.* 6, 78–83.

Schuurman, A.G., Goldbohm, R.A., Dorant, E., and van den Brandt, P.A. (1998). Vegetable and fruit consumption and prostate cancer risk: A cohort study in The Netherlands. *Cancer Epidemiol. Biomarkers Prev.* 7, 673–680.

Schwartz, A.G., Hard, G.C., Pashko, L.L., Abou–Gharbia, M., and Swern, D. (1981). Dehydroepiandrosterone: An anti-obesity and anti-carcinogenic agent. *Nutr. Cancer* 3.

Schwetz, B.A. (2001). Safety of aristolochic acid. *JAMA* 285, 2705.

Science Advisory Board (2001). *An SAB Report: Review of the Office of Research and Development's Reassessment of Dioxin*. US Environmental Protection Agency, Washington, DC.

Sellers, T.A., Bazyk, A.E., Bostick, R.M., Kushi, L.H., Olson, J.E., Anderson, K.E., Lazovich, D., and Folsom, A.R. (1998). Diet and risk of colon cancer in a large prospective study of older women: An analysis stratified on family history (Iowa, United States). *Cancer Causes Control* 9, 357–367.

Sen, N.P., Seaman, S., and Miles, W.F. (1979). Volatile nitrosamines in various cured meat products: Effect of cooking and recent trends. *J. Agric. Food Chem.* 27, 1354–1357.

Senti, F.R., and Pilch, S.M. (1985). Analysis of folate data from the second National Health and Nutrition Examination Survey (NHANES II). *J. Nutr.* 115, 1398–1402.

Setchell, K.D., Zimmer-Nechemias, L., Cai, J., and Heubi, J.E. (1997). Exposure of infants to phyto-oestrogens from soy-based infant formula. *Lancet* 350, 23–27.

Shacter, E., Beecham, E.J., Covey, J.M., Kohn, K.W., and Potter, M. (1988). Activated neutrophils induce prolonged DNA damage in neighboring cells. *Carcinogenesis* 9, 2297–2304. [published erratum appears in *Carcinogenesis* 10: 628 (1989)].

Shields, P.G., Xu, G.X., Blot, W.J., Fraumeni, J.F., Jr., Trivers, G.E., Pellizzari, E.D., Qu, Y.H., Gao, Y.T., and Harris, C.C. (1995). Mutagens from heated Chinese and US cooking oils. *J. Natl. Cancer Inst.* 87, 836–841.

Siegal, D.M., Frankos, V.H., and Schneiderman, M. (1983). Formaldehyde risk assessment for occupationally exposed workers. *Reg. Toxicol. Pharm.* 3, 355–371.

Smiciklas-Wright, H., Mitchell, D.C., Mickle, S.J., Cook, A.J., and Goldman, J.D. (2002). *Foods Commonly Eaten in the United States: Quantities Consumed per Eating Occasion and in a Day, 1994–1996*. US Department of Agriculture, Beltsville, MD. http://www.barc.usda.gov/bhnrc/foodsurvey/pdf/Portion.pdf.

Smith, R.L., Adams, T.B., Doull, J., Feron, V.J., Goodman, J.I., Marnett, L.J., Protoghese, P.S., Waddell, W.J., Wagner, B.M., Rogers, A.E., Caldwell, J., and Sipes, I.G. (2002). Safety assessment of allylalkoxybenzene derivatives used as flavouring substances—methyl eugenol and estragole. *Food Chem. Toxicol.* 40, 851–870.

Smith-Warner, S.A., Spiegelman, D., Yaun, S.S., Adami, H.O., Beeson, W.L., van den Brandt, P.A., Folsom,

A.R., Fraser, G.E., Freudenheim, J.L., Goldbohm, R.A., Graham, S., Miller, A.B., Potter, J.D., Rohan, T.E., Speizer, F.E., Toniolo, P., Willett, W.C., Wolk, A., Zeleniuch-Jacquotte, A., and Hunter, D.J. (2001). Intake of fruits and vegetables and risk of breast cancer: a pooled analysis of cohort studies. *JAMA* 285, 769–776.

Snyderwine, E.g., Turesky, R.J., Turteltaub, K.W., Davis, C.D., Sadrieh, N., Schut, H.A.J., Nagao, M., Sugimura, T., Thorgeirsson, U.P., Adamson, R.H., and Snorri, S. (1997). Metabolism of food-derived heterocyclic amines in nonhuman primates. *Mutat. Res.* 376, 203–210.

Sorahan, T., Lancashire, S., Prior, P., Peck, I., and Stewart, A. (1995). Childhood cancer and parental use of alcohol and tobacco. *Ann. Epidemiol.* 5, 354–359.

Starr, T.B. (2001). Significant shortcomings of the US Environmental Protection Agency's latest draft risk characterization for dioxin-like compounds. *Toxicol Sci* 64, 7–13.

Steinmetz, K.A., and Potter, J.D. (1996). Vegetables, fruit, and cancer prevention: A review. *J. Am. Diet. Assoc.* 96, 1027–1039.

Stickel, F., and Seitz, H.K. (2000). The efficacy and safety of comfrey. *Pub. Health Nutr.* 3, 501–508.

Stofberg, J., and Grundschober, F. (1987). Consumption ratio and food predominance of flavoring materials. Second cumulative series. *Perfum. Flavor.* 12, 27–56.

Stöhr, H., and Herrmann, K. (1975). Über die Phenolsäuren des Gemüses: III. Hydroxyzimtsäuren und Hydroxybenzoesäuren des Wurzelgemüses. *Z. Lebensm. Unters. Forsch.* 159, 219–224.

Stoll, B.A. (1999). Dietary supplements of dehydroepiandrosterone in relation to breast cancer risk. *Eur. J. Clin. Nutr.* 53, 771–775.

Subar, A.F., Block, G., and James, L.D. (1989). Folate intake and food sources in the US population. *Am. J. Clin. Nutr.* 50, 508–516.

Swan, S.H., Elkin, E.P., and Fenster, L. (1997). Have sperm densities declined? A reanalysis of global trend data. *Environ. Health Perspect.* 105, 1228–1232. Letters: 106: A370–371, A420–421.

Swenberg, J.A., and Lehman–McKeeman, L.D. (1999). α_{2u}-Urinary globulin-associated nephropathy as a mechanism of renal tubule cell carcinogenesis in male rats. In *Species Differences in Thyroid, Kidney and Urinary Bladder Carcinogenesis* (C.C. Capen, E. Dybing, J.M. Rice and J.D. Wilbourn, eds.), Vol. 147, pp. 95–118. International Agency for Research on Cancer, Lyon, France.

Takahashi, S., Tamano, S., Hirose, M., Kimoto, N., Ikeda, Y., Sakakibara, M., Tada, M., Kadlubar, F.F., Ito, N., and Shirai, T. (1998). Immunohistochemical demonstration of carcinogen-DNA adducts in tissues of rats given 2-amino-1-methyl-6-phenylimidazo[4,5-b]pyridine (PhIP): detection in paraffin–embedded sections and tissue distribution. *Cancer Res.* 58, 4307–4313.

Takayama, S., Sieber, S.M., Adamson, R.H., Thorgeirsson, U.P., Dalgard, D.W., Arnold, L.L., Cano, M., Eklund, S., and Cohen, S.M. (1998). Long-term feeding of sodium saccharin to nonhuman primates: Implications for urinary tract cancer. *J. Natl. Cancer Inst.* 90, 19–25.

Takayama, S., Sieber, S.M., Dalgard, D.W., Thorgeirsson, U.P., and Adamson, R.H. (1999). Effects of long-term oral administration of DDT on nonhuman primates. *J. Cancer Res. Clin. Oncol.* 125, 219–225.

Tareke, E., Rydberg, P., Karlsson, P., Eriksson, S., and Törnqvist, M. (2002). Analysis of acrylamide, a carcinogen formed in heated foodstuffs. *J. Agric. Food Chem.* 50, 4998–5006.

Technical Assessment Systems (1989). *Exposure 1 Software Package.* TAS, Washington, DC. Provided by Barbara Petersen.

Tengs, T.O., Adams, M.E., Pliskin, J.S., Safran, D.G., Siegel, J.E., Weinstein, M.C., and Graham, J.D. (1995). Five-hundred life-saving interventions and their cost-effectiveness. *Risk Anal.* 15, 369–390.

Terry, P., Nyrén, O., and Yuen, J. (1998). Protective effect of fruits and vegetables on stomach cancer in a cohort of Swedish twins. *Int. J. Cancer* 76, 35–37.

Terry, P., Suzuki, R., Hu, F.B., and Wolk, A. (2001). A prospective study of major dietary patterns and the risk of breast cancer. *Cancer Epidemiol. Biomarkers Prev.* 10, 1281–1285.

Theranaturals (2000). *Theranaturals I3C Caps.* http://www.theranaturals.com/.

Thorgeirsson, U.P., Dalgard, D.W., Reeves, J., and Adamson, R.H. (1994). Tumor incidence in a chemical carcinogenesis study in nonhuman primates. *Regul. Toxicol. Pharmacol.* 19, 130–151.

Tomatis, L., and Bartsch, H. (1990). The contribution of experimental studies to risk assessment of carcinogenic agents in humans. *Exp. Pathol.* 40, 251–266.

Toth, B., and Erickson, J. (1986). Cancer induction in mice by feeding of the uncooked cultivated mushroom of commerce *Agaricus bisporus. Cancer Res.* 46, 4007–4011.

Tressl, R. (1976). Aromastoffe des Bieres und Ihre Entstehung. *Brauwelt Jg.* 39, 1252–1259.

Tressl, R., Bahri, D., Köppler, H., and Jensen, A. (1978). Diphenole und Caramelkomponenten in Röstkaffees verschiedener Sorten. II. *Z. Lebensm. Unters. Forsch.* 167, 111–114.

Tricker, A.R., and Preussmann, R. (1991). Carcinogenic N–nitrosamines in the diet: Occurrence, formation, mechanisms and carcinogenic potential. *Mutat. Res.* 259, 277–289.

Trosko, J.E. (1998). Hierarchical and cybernetic nature of biologic systems and their relevance to homeostatic adaptation to low-level exposures to oxidative stress-inducing agents. *Environ. Health Perspect.* 106 (Suppl. 1), 331–339.

Tsao, R., Yu, Q., Potter, J., and Chiba, M. (2002). Direct and simultaneous analysis of sinigrin and allyl isothiocyanate in mustard samples by high–performance liquid chromatography. *J. Agric. Food Chem.* 50, 4749–4753.

Turturro, A., Duffy, P., Hart, R., and Allaben, W.T. (1996). Rationale for the use of dietary control in toxicity studies-B6C3F$_1$ mouse. *Toxicol. Pathol.* 24, 769–775.

US Department of Agriculture (2000). *United States: Imports of Specified Condiments, Seasonings, and Flavor Materials by Country of Origin.* USDA, Washington, DC.

US Department of Heath and Human Services (1986). *The Health Consequences of Involuntary Smoking: A Report of the Surgeon General.* USDHHS, Rockville, MD.

US Environmental Protection Agency (1987). *Peer Review of Chlorothalonil.* Office of Pesticides and Toxic Substances, Washington, DC. Review found in Health Effect Division Document No. 007718.

US Environmental Protection Agency (1991a). *EBDC/ETU Special Review. DRES Dietary Exposure/Risk Estimates.* USEPA, Washington, DC. Memo from R. Griffin to K. Martin.

US Environmental Protection Agency (1991b). *Environmental Investments: The Cost of a Clean Environment.* USEPA, Washington, DC.

US Environmental Protection Agency (1991c). *Report of the EPA Peer Review Workshop on Alpha$_{2u}$-globulin: Association with Renal Toxicity and Neoplasia in the Male Rat.* USEPA, Washington, DC.

US Environmental Protection Agency (1992a). Ethylene bisdithiocarbamates (EBDCs); Notice of intent to cancel; Conclusion of special review. *Fed. Reg.* 57, 7484–7530.

US Environmental Protection Agency (1992b). *Respiratory Health Effects of Passive Smoking: Lung Cancer and Other Disorders.* USEPA, Washington, DC. EPA/660/6–90/006F.

US Environmental Protection Agency (1994a). *Estimating Exposure to Dioxin-Like Compounds (Review Draft).* USEPA, Washington, DC.

US Environmental Protection Agency (1994b). *Health Assessment Document for 2,3,7,8-Tetrachlorodibenzo-p-Dioxin (TCDD) and Related Compounds.* USEPA, Washington, DC.

US Environmental Protection Agency (1995). *Re–evaluating Dioxin: Science Advisory Board's Review of EPA's Reassessment of Dioxin and Dioxin–Like Compounds.* USEPA, Washington, DC.

US Environmental Protection Agency (1997). *Exposure Factors Handbook.* USEPA, Washington, DC.

US Environmental Protection Agency (1998a). *Assessment of Thyroid Follicular Cell Tumors.* USEPA, Washington, DC.

US Environmental Protection Agency (1998b). *Status of Pesticides in Registration, Reregistration, and Special Review.* USEPA, Washington, DC.

US Environmental Protection Agency (1999). *Draft Revised Guidelines for Carcinogen Risk Assessment.* USEPA, Washington, DC.

US Environmental Protection Agency (2000). *Exposure and Human Health Reassessment of 2,3,7,8-Tetrachlorodibenzo-p-Dioxin (TCDD) and Related Compounds. Draft Final.* USEPA, Washington, DC.

US Environmental Protection Agency (2001). *Dioxin: Summary of the Dioxin Reassessment Science, Information Sheet 1.* USEPA, Washington, DC.

US Environmental Protection Agency (2002). *Integrated Risk Information System (IRIS).* Office of Health and Environmental Assessment, Environmental Criteria and Assessment Office, Cincinnati, OH.

US Environmental Protection Agency. Office of Pesticide Programs (February 8, 1984). *Ethylene Dibromide (EDB) Scientific Support and Decision Document for Grain and Grain Milling Fumigation Uses.* USEPA, Washington, DC.

US Environmental Protection Agency. Office of Pesticide Programs (1989). *Daminozide Special Review. Technical Support Document—Preliminary Determination to Cancel the Food Uses of Daminozide.* USEPA, Washington, DC.

US Food and Drug Administration (1960). Refusal to extend effective date of statute for certain specified additives in food. *Fed. Reg.* 25, 12412.

US Food and Drug Administration (1991a). *Butylatedhydroxyanisole (BHA) Intake: Memo from Food and Additives Color Section to L. Lin.* USFDA, Washington, DC.

US Food and Drug Administration (1991b). FDA Pesticide Program: Residues in foods 1990. *J. Assoc. Off. Anal. Chem.* 74, 121A–141A.

US Food and Drug Administration (1992). *Exposure to Aflatoxins.* Food and Drug Administration, Washington, DC.

US Food and Drug Administration (1993a). *Assessment of Carcinogenic Upper Bound Lifetime Risk from Resulting Aflatoxins in Consumer Peanut and Corn Products. Report of the Quantitative Risk Assessment Committee.* USFDA, Washington, DC.

US Food and Drug Administration (1993b). Food and Drug Administration Pesticide Program: Residue monitoring 1992. *J. Assoc. Off. Anal. Chem.* 76, 127A–148A.

US Food and Drug Administration (2002). *Mushroom Promotion, Research, and Consumer Information Order, Vol. 2002.* US FDA. http://www.ams.usda.gov/fv/rpmushroom.html.

US National Cancer Institute (1996). Why eat five? *J. Natl. Cancer Inst.* 88, 1314.

US National Toxicology Program (1998). *Fiscal Year 1998 Annual Plan.* DHHS, Public Health Service, National Institutes of Health, Washington, DC. http://ntpserver.niehs.nih.gov/htdocs/98AP/contents.html.

US National Toxicology Program (2000a). *Background Information Indole-3-carbinol (I3C) 700-06-1.* NTP, Research Triangle Park, NC. http://ntpserver.niehs.nih.gov/htdocs/Chem_Background/ExSumPdf/Indolecarbinol.pdf.

US National Toxicology Program (2000b). *Ninth Report on Carcinogens.* NTP, Research Triangle Park, NC.

US National Toxicology Program (2001). *Addendum to Ninth Report on Carcinogens: 2,3,7,8-Tetrachlorodibenzo-p-Dioxin (TCDD); DIOXIN CAS No. 1746–01–6.* NTP, Research Triangle Park, NC.

Van den Berg, M., Birnbaum, L., Bosveld, A.T., Brunstrom, B., Cook, P., Feeley, M., Giesy, J.P., Hanberg, A., Hasegawa, R., Kennedy, S.W., Kubiak, T., Larsen, J.C., van Leeuwen, F.X., Liem, A.K., Nolt, C., Peterson, R.E., Poellinger, L., Safe, S., Schrenk, D., Tillitt, D., Tysklind, M., Younes, M., Waern, F., and Zacharewski, T. (1998). Toxic equivalency factors (TEFs) for PCBs, PCDDs, PCDFs for humans and wildlife. *Environ Health Perspect* 106, 775–792.

Vainio, H., and Bianchini, F., eds. (2002). *Weight Control and Physical Activity.* IARC Press, Lyon, France.

Vainio, H., Wilbourn, J.D., Sasco, A.J., Partensky, C., Gaudin, N., Heseltine, E., and Eragne, I. (1995). Identification des facteurs cancérogènes pour l'homme dans les Monographies du CIRC. *Bull. Cancer* 82, 339–348.

van Vollenhoven, R.F. (2000). Dehydroepiandrosterone in systemic lupus erythematosus. *Rheum. Dis. Clin. North. Am.* 26, 339–348.

Viscusi, W.K. (1992). *Fatal Tradeoffs: Public & Private Responsibilities for Risk.* Oxford University Press, New York.

Volpe, J. (1998). *Natural Health Products: A New Vision, Vol. 2001*. Health Canada. http://www.parl.gc.ca/InfoComDoc/36/1/HEAL/Studies/Reports/healrp02-e.htm.

Voorrips, L.E., Goldbohm, R.A., van Poppel, G., Sturmans, F., Hermus, R.J.J., and van den Brandt, P.A. (2000). Vegetable and fruit consumption and risks of colon and rectal cancer in a prospective cohort study. *Am. J. Epidemiol.* 152, 1081–1092.

Wallock, L.M., Tamura, T., Mayr, C.A., Johnston, K.E., Ames, B.N., and Jacob, R.A. (2001). Low seminal plasma folate concentrations are associated with low sperm density and count in male smokers and nonsmokers. *Fertil. Steril.* 75, 252–259.

Wei, L., Wei, H., and Frenkel, K. (1993a). Sensitivity to tumor promotion of SENCAR and C57Bl/6J mice correlates with oxidative events and DNA damage. *Carcinogenesis* 14, 841–847.

Wei, Q., Matanoski, G.M., Farmer, E.R., Hedayati, M.A., and Grossman, L. (1993b). DNA repair and aging in basal cell carcinoma: A molecular epidemiology study [published erratum appears in Proc. Natl. Acad. Sci. USA 1993 Jun 1;90(11):5378]. *Proc. Natl. Acad. Sci. USA* 90, 1614–1618.

Wheeler, R.E., Pragnell, M.J., and Pierce, J.S. (1971). The identificaiton of factors affecting flavour stability in beer. *Eur. Brew. Conv. Proc. Cong.* 1971, 423–436.

Wildavsky, A.B. (1988). *Searching for Safety*. Transaction Books, New Brunswick, NJ.

Wildavsky, A.B. (1995). *But Is It True? A Citizen's Guide to Environmental Health and Safety Issues*. Harvard University Press, Cambridge, MA.

Wilker, C., Johnson, L., and Safe, S. (1996). Effects of developmental exposure to indole-3-carbinol or 2,3,7,8-tetrachlorodibenzo-*p*-dioxin on reproductive potential of male rat offspring. *Toxicol. Appl. Pharmacol.* 141, 68–75.

Willett, W.C. (2001). Diet and cancer: One view at the start of the millennium. *Cancer Epidemiol. Biomarkers Prev.* 10, 3–8.

Wine Institute (2001). *Per Capita Wine Consumption in Selected Countries, Vol. 2002.* Wine Institute. http://www.wineinstitute.org/communications/statistics/keyfacts_worldpercapitaconsumption01.htm.

Woodall, A.A., and Ames, B.N. (1997). Diet and oxidative damage to DNA: The importance of ascorbate as an antioxidant. In *Vitamin C in Health and Disease* (L. Packer, ed.), pp. 193–203. Marcel Dekker, New York.

World Cancer Research Fund (1997). *Food, Nutrition and the Prevention of Cancer: A Global Perspective.* American Institute for Cancer Research, Washington, DC.

World Health Organization (1984). WHO cooperative trial on primary prevention of ischaemic heart disease with clofibrate to lower serum cholesterol: final mortality follow–up. Report of the Committee of Principal Investigators. *Lancet* 8403, 600–604.

World Health Organization (1993). *Polychlorinated Biphenyls and Terphenyls.* WHO, Geneva.

Writing Group for the Women's Health Initiative Investigators (2002). Risks and benefits of estrogen plus progestin in healthy postmenopausal women. Principal results from the Women's Health Initiative randomized controlled trial. *JAMA* 288, 321–333.

Wu–Williams, A.H., Zeise, L., and Thomas, D. (1992). Risk assessment for aflatoxin B_1: A modeling approach. *Risk Anal.* 12, 559–567.

Wyrobek, A.J., Rubes, J., Cassel, M., Moore, D., Perrault, S., Slott, V., Evenson, D., Zudova, Z., Borkovec, L., Selevan, S., and Lowe, X. (1995). Smokers produce more aneuploid sperm than non–smokers. *Am. J. Hum. Genet.* 57 (Suppl.), A131.

Yamashina, K., Miller, B.E., and Heppner, G.H. (1986). Macrophage-mediated induction of drug-resistant variants in a mouse mammary tumor cell line. *Cancer Res.* 46, 2396–2401.

Yu, M.C., Tong, M.J., Govindarajan, S., and Henderson, B.E. (1991). Nonviral risk factors for hepatocellular carcinoma in a low-risk population, the non-Asians of Los Angeles County, California. *J. Natl. Cancer Inst.* 83, 1820–1826.

Zeegers, M.P.A., Goldbohm, R.A., and van den Brandt, P.A. (2001). Consumption of vegetables and fruits and urothelial cancer incidence: A prospective study. *Cancer Epidemiol. Biomarkers Prev.* 10, 1121–1128.

Zhang, J.Z., Henning, S.M., and Swendseid, M.E. (1993). Poly(ADP-ribose) polymerase activity and DNA strand breaks are affected in tissues of niacin-deficient rats. *J. Nutr.* 123, 1349–1355.